FAT ◆TO◆ FANTASTIC

Denise Taylor was once told off by her boss for being like Pollyanna and took it as a compliment. She lives in the Gloucestershire countryside with her husband Simon. She is a Chartered Psychologist, Associate Fellow of the British Psychological Society and a double award winning career coach with Amazing People (www.amazingpeople.co.uk) a bespoke career consultancy, small from choice. You will learn much more about Denise as you read through this book.

Articles by Denise are regularly featured in print and online and she is a regular contributor to radio shows where she discusses a wide range of topics related to careers, job searching and motivation.

Ambitions include completing a trip to Antarctica, DJing at a festival, trekking to Everest Base Camp and ultimately being able to look back on her life, knowing she made a difference to others, inspiring them to be fit and healthy.

Brook House Press
www.brookhousepress.com
simon@brookhousepress.com

Disclaimer:

This book is not intended to take the place of medical advice from a trained medical professional. We recommend you contact a doctor or qualified health professional before making any changes to your diet or embarking upon any exercise regime. Neither the publisher nor the author take any responsibility for any possible consequences that may arise as a result of following the information in this book.

ISBN 978-0-9561755-2-6

Cover and Interior Design by Tudor Maier

Further information can be found at www.FAT2fantastic.com

By the same author

How to Get a Job in a Recession 2012, 2nd edition, Brook House Press
Now You've Been Shortlisted, Harriman House
Winning Interview Answers for First-time Job Hunters, Trotman Publishing
How to Get a Job in a Recession, 1st edition, Brook House Press
17th Century Wedding Customs (Living History Reference Books), Stuart Press

FAT ◆ FANTASTIC

**An Inspirational Diary of Middle Aged Weight Loss,
Based on Healthy Eating, Regular Exercise and Masses of
Drive and Determination**

How I lost over 10 stone in weight and found my confident fun loving self

By Denise Taylor

Brook House Press
www.brookhousepress.com
simon@brookhousepress.com

CONTENTS

INTRODUCTION FROM SIMON
THE HUSBAND

I am so proud of my wife. To be honest I never thought she would do it, she has moaned about being fat, gone on diets and then gone off them. With each diet I've thought 'here we go again', she got stroppy from lack of food, gave up and ate rich food, then got upset when she realised she had failed again.

She is such a motivated and determined woman but this was the area of her life that was out of control, she seemed to be able to eat and eat and couldn't say no. Chocolate was the worst, when she was on a diet she'd still phone me at work to bring some chocolate home as she felt stressed and if I didn't I'd have to go out again. It was so hard, knowing that it wasn't doing her any good at all. I really was worried about her health!

I also felt sorry for her. Now I love her to bits but as we walked out in public I'd notice how people would look at her, especially young women who would point at and talk about the fat woman. She never noticed, I don't think she would look at people but I noticed and it was sad. In midlife you don't really get looked at, but she was getting unwelcome attention.

It did take her four years but by her 50th birthday she had lost six and a half stone so was looking much better, but then following a holiday in Namibia where we ended up eating a lot of stodgy food, the weight went back on. I tried to support her to lose weight, but I don't think me saying *do you think you should have that?*' was making much difference. I tried to be supportive but you can't convince someone else to do something.

Over the next couple of years she put three stone back on - I kept trying to encourage her but she would say that she wanted chocolate, it was almost always chocolate or ice cream and it is hard to say no to someone you love when they look at you with pleading eyes like a fat Labrador wanting a snack.

I was worried about how this affected her work as a careers coach, what must her clients think of her? She had tried meal replacements but that wasn't satisfying, she wanted proper food.

She hadn't got on the scales for months, and when, in early October she got on the scales and weighed in at 18 stone 13 I didn't expect this time to be different. This would be another two weeks of being very disciplined and then giving up. This time, however, she said she was committed and met up with a personal trainer, Ben Carpenter. I still didn't have much faith, I'd heard it all before. But this time it was different. She started telling people, writing on her blog and on Facebook and listening to Ben. She ate what he told her to and she started to do serious exercise.

I'm now so proud of her. She has done so well and I can't stop looking at my new wife, she looks so good! It's great to go clothes shopping with her, it's no longer the miserable experience it was because she can now buy things that she looks good in.

Previously she would never look in the mirror and would pull away if I went to touch her, now she likes to be touched and is far more confident in her body.

I always loved Denise but I really love the new Denise, I really am so proud of her.

Simon Taylor
Proud Husband

INTRODUCTION FROM EMMA
THE PERSONAL TRAINER

I have been a trainer at Denise's gym for many, many years and have seen her start her attempt to lose weight, make progress, struggle and fail several times and it's been heartbreaking because inside that fat person (and yes, she was fat, she'll be the first to admit it!) was a slim, happy one trying so hard to get out!

It was as if fate had stepped in the day she found Ben; he was the perfect trainer for her at the time and we saw a different Denise coming into the gym; I remember the change, instead of sidling in head down she'd march in, programme tucked under her elbow, bottle of water gripped in her hand with a determination in her face we'd not seen before! I watched from the sidelines as Ben battered her all over the gym and she took it, she worked hard with Ben and even harder on her own and I saw her literally melt away before my eyes. I remember one day she walked through the door and I had to give her a huge hug and say how proud not only Ben, but every other Trainer at the gym was of her, of her dedication, her commitment and her drive. This person was changing in front of us, cheeky little smiles started to appear where as before she'd simply try and melt into the background; the confidence was coming back as the pounds dropped off. And heck it has to be said, what a butt! Ben did an amazing job with Denise, he spotted her insulin resistance issue, prescribed the appropriate diet and supplementation and gave her big weights to lump around, and she did it all, every single thing he asked of her she did. That's Denise all over really, she's an all or nothing kinda gal!

Unfortunately Ben had to leave our Gym for personal reasons and believe me if you've ever had a trainer then you'll know that losing them is like having a rug pulled from under you but Denise didn't falter and fortunately for me I had built up a rapport with Denise over her time with Ben and knew I could help her continue her journey. I was delighted when she decided to keep up her training with me. By this time she'd lost an enormous amount of weight so lucky me got her when it was hardest, the less you have to lose the harder it becomes! And boy have we been through some ups, some downs, I've yelled at her at times, kicked her up the butt, begged, pleaded, beasted her, watched in disbelief as injury after injury slowed her down but together we have found ways around things because if you want something bad enough you will do exactly what Denise has done, you will GO OUT AND GET IT! It was so frustrating for me as her Trainer (and now a good friend) to see her start to lose focus when she was sooooooo close to her goal ... it was after a significant bit of yo-yoing that I decided enough was enough, that it was time to mix it up a bit and to turn Denise's world upside down by changing her diet completely by BRINGING BACK CARBS! I thought she was going to have a coronary but just like always, her desire to be the best meant she embraced the change (with only minor moaning!), and now I have my bouncy, cheerful, energetic maniac back, the one that trains like a demon, makes me laugh like a drain and is one of the most amazing people I have ever met. A pleasure to train and an inspiration to all.

Read on, it is a tale of highs, lows, facts and tips, bits in between, laughs and more. If it doesn't inspire you to do what you need to do then maybe you need a kick up the butt too!

Be Loud, Be Proud Denise, your achievement is undeniable and we all love you for it!

Emma Brace
Master Personal Trainer & Sports Massage Therapist

I've missed more than 9000 shots in my career. I've lost almost 300 games. 26 times, I've been trusted to take the game winning shot and missed. I've failed over and over and over again in my life. And that is why I succeed.

— *Michael Jordan*

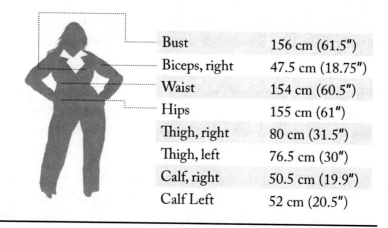

Bust	156 cm (61.5")
Biceps, right	47.5 cm (18.75")
Waist	154 cm (60.5")
Hips	155 cm (61")
Thigh, right	80 cm (31.5")
Thigh, left	76.5 cm (30")
Calf, right	50.5 cm (19.9")
Calf Left	52 cm (20.5")

I once weighed 22.5 stone and got down to 15 stone 12 (a huge loss of more than 6.5 stone) but then I went on holiday, stopped eating sensibly and the weight crept back up. However, on the plus side, I'm still 50lb lighter than I was at my fattest. I hate the word fat but it's the right way to describe how I looked. Of course, my weight alone doesn't define me as a person, but people make judgements all the time based on appearance.

In the past, I've tried them all - Rosemary Conley, Weight Watchers, Cambridge Diet, Cabbage Soup Diet, Slimming World, Herbalife.

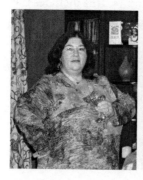
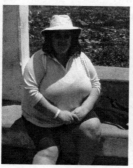
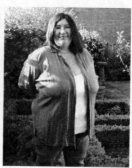

They all worked to some extent but the group programmes weren't for me and I like eating. The best was probably a meal replacement programme swapping shakes for 2 meals a day and I did lose 6 stone 9lb with this. I think it was the weekly phone calls that were motivational and the insistence that I ate lots of colour (salads, fruit, and veggies) but eventually I got bored of meal replacement shakes and craved 'real' food.

Why did I allow the weight to pile on again? It's a rhetorical question, I know the answer, I ate too much, didn't do enough exercise and enjoyed my food and drink more than the thought of being slim and looking good in my clothes.

I loved food, I loved the feeling of being full, I hated being hungry. I saw food as my friend and used food to comfort me. I've had stress in my life and food helped to block out the pain. I used food to sedate myself from painful thoughts and it also gave me a lot of pleasure. I loved the feeling of chocolate melting down my throat, much more my thing than the salty taste of savoury snacks. I overcame all of this, however, and eventually I reached my goal.

ADDICTED TO FOOD

Food was an addiction to me but unlike alcoholics and smokers I can't avoid food. It was not my choice to be fat. What I learned was that my body was starving - craving nutrients - and that's why I ate so much.

I know the things that only a really fat person knows. This includes the shame of having to ask for a seat belt extension on the plane, the horror of the man sat next to me asking to be moved away from the 'grande dame' (I knew enough French to know what he was saying). I've felt the embarrassment of swimming, knowing I looked like a whale and of discovering that not even a large bath sheet would meet when I put it around my body.

When you are fat, you tend to forget about the horrible embarrassing experiences. One time I went to a crematorium to celebrate the life of a dear friend who died. Another car parked so close to mine that I couldn't get into the car. I had to ask someone else to get into the car and reverse it out so I could get in and drive away. It's no wonder I hide memories like this in the back of my mind.

HOW FAT PEOPLE WALK

Have you ever watched a fat person walk down the street? There's a particular sound we make as our thighs rub together. We don't want to be seen so we have our head down, we try to make ourselves as small as possible so we have our arms by our sides. We also dress in black, there is no colour in our clothes and there was little colour in my life when I was huge.

I took massive action. I kept this diary both to chart progress and to motivate myself, and now you.

I'm assuming you've picked up this book because, as I was, you are fed up of being fat and getting worried about your health. I was at high risk of diabetes, heart disease and more. At 18 stone 13 I was still morbidly obese; at 22.5 stone I was heading for an early death.

This book tells you what I did and I can assure you that my results didn't come easily. I've had days that I wanted to give up and eat a big chunk of crusty bread and cheese or a glass or 3 of wine. For the first 6 months I kept focused on the end goal. I thought I had been highly focused and only went off plan on the days I was told I could have a 'carb meal'. However, reading through my diary, I can see that I wasn't always 100% faithful to the plan but thankfully I was faithful enough overall. I let up a bit later on, and my progress slowed down, but I needed to make my eating and exercise plan part of my life for it to be sustainable once I'd reached my final goal.

The food plan I followed was low carb. It's not the only way to lose weight but a lot of evidence states that people with a lot of weight to lose are insulin resistant. Eating lots of vegetables in addition to protein is an excellent way to lose weight, and more importantly, to get healthier and reduce the risk of diabetes.

INSULIN RESISTANT

This means that when carbs are turned into glycogen in the blood, instead of letting insulin push it through into the muscles where it can be used as energy, the muscles block the process and insulin then stores the glycogen as fat. Being overweight and sedentary causes this because our muscles aren't working efficiently. This state of affairs can be changed with exercise so you can then eat carbs.

I have not been 100% good all the time, but what changed this time was that if I really fancied something - Waitrose Vanilla cheesecake - yummy, yumm! - I would eat it and enjoy it. I used to have this voice in my head that told me that if I ate it quickly it wouldn't count. Maybe you have such voices too. I know that this is clearly not true and if you are going to eat something you should really enjoy it, savouring every mouthful, but I have learnt you can't be a healthy weight if you have treats every day and you really do need to increase activity levels regardless.

This book is not the story of a quick fix, it's a story of struggle and perseverance. By January 2010, I weighed 12 stone 03lbs. This may sound a bit heavy but I have built a lot of muscle. I then spent over a year gaining and losing the same 7lb or so, just like everyone else. I kept up the exercise, however, and eventually regained my focus for a final push to crack the 12 stone barrier. Whilst I struggled I felt like a failure, wondering why I wasn't losing the weight, but as I read all my notes when writing this book it became clear why I didn't lose the weight. I put the short term satisfaction of eating food I love above my health goals. Reading my diary re-motivated me and I hope it will motivate you.

My new goal is to motivate others to lose the unhealthy fat and find their fit and healthy selves. I don't want people to be skinny minxes but I do want them to enjoy life and feel uplifted by the energy we get from looking after ourselves and making good choices most of the time.

I'm now 54, 5'5" and happily married to Simon. We married 14 years ago, a second marriage for us both, and our children have grown and now have their own independent lives. Now that I am fit and healthy again the world is my oyster and I look forward to what it brings. I've rediscovered the joy of life.

I really hope you enjoy this book and I would love to hear how you get on.

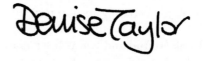

Denise Taylor
December 2011
Tewkesbury, England

www.fat2fantastic.com
www.facebook.com/Fat2Fantastic
twitter.com/fat2fantastic

It's my personal opinion that the diet industry wants to keep us fat. Globally, it's a multi billion pound industry after all and it would collapse if we stopped buying their products. Why do slimming clubs encourage us to buy their diet snacks and processed foods rather than fruit and veg? Because of the profit they can make from these products. Food manufacturers are more interested in selling us processed food with a higher profit margin than encouraging us to eat natural food. There's not much profit in selling a potato, but much more when that potato can be cheaply processed into an expensive packet of crisps.

Processed food and sugar is addictive. When we snack on a can of cola (including diet cola) there's a high amount of sugar or sugar substitute, chocolate is high in fat, etc. These lead to a spike in blood sugar which results in us being hungry about an hour later and also sets us on the track to becoming insulin resistant.

Look around and you will see many people with a high amount of fat around their middle, this belly fat is quite a new phenomenon. From what I've read it is attributable to the type of food people eat - highly processed. It can also be caused by a lack of sleep and stress.

Conflicting advice - who do you believe?

I'm not a dietician but I am a chartered psychologist and I like to research. I've read extensively on what does and doesn't work and used this to help me to lose a substantial amount of weight. I still have to pinch myself to remind myself that I really have lost over 10.5 stone!

One thing I've learnt through my research is that you need to think about why certain information is being shared. Newspapers and magazines write to sell copies and they know that details on the latest diet leads to more sales. They usually offer quick fixes rather than sensible nutritional advice because people want to believe the battle can be won easily! Experts can also get things wrong, some dieticians advise diabetics to eat carbs whereas my understanding is that they need to be on a low carb diet to reduce their insulin response.

The need to care for yourself

Many people overeat because they value themselves the least. We spend too much time looking after everyone else and we forget about us, so we snatch a bite to eat that's quick and our choices are often not great. Often, we are hungry for calm and balance and we need this as much as food. We have to prioritise and place our own well being higher on our list, taking time out to enjoy the foods which will nourish us.

Emotional eating

Many times we eat to meet our emotional needs. We eat because we are experiencing boredom, frustration, anger, loneliness or depression. In the short term, food can help to deal with the emotion but in the longer term we have the additional problem of weight gain. Most of us don't realise that overeating is a form of self harm - when we eat more than we need, or want, we are hurting our body.

PSYCHOLOGY OF WEIGHT LOSS

Losing weight is partly down to exercise and healthy eating but also down to what goes on in our heads, our inner monologue. As a morbidly obese psychologist I knew this but it took commitment to my goal of becoming fit and healthy before I applied what I knew to my own life and approach.

It is in my nature to find out as much as I can on a subject. I love to learn and so to enhance what I already knew I studied sports and exercise psychology (and gained a distinction!). This was very helpful in revisiting topics such as imagery and goal setting from a different perspective. I also read extensively, going beyond popular books to scientific research to ensure what I was doing was based on what works. *My focus was on health, not weight loss. A focus on health would lead to weight loss but a focus on weight loss could have lead to poor food choices.*

Loving not loathing

Being overweight is not the only way to describe ourselves. It's just one part of who we are. We are also kind, interesting, determined, curious ... and in my case I am also a mother, sister, daughter and friend.

We need to love ourselves for who we are right now instead of just thinking everything will be better in the future. We need to care for ourselves and treat ourselves well. When we don't like ourselves we don't treat ourselves well because we don't think we deserve such treatment. So, if we really want to have a bar of chocolate, we should buy good quality high cocoa chocolate and take the time to savour it properly. We should sit down, open the packaging slowly, smell it and really take in the aroma, break off just one square and enjoy the full taste. Far better to enjoy it than to cram it into our mouth, disgusted with ourselves.

Motivation - why do we want to lose weight?

Motivation can be internally generated or externally generated. We can do something because our partner wants us to, or a doctor advises us to, but it's hard to keep going when a goal is based on external factors.

Different things motivate us. We are either motivated to go towards something or motivated to pull away from it and achieving a goal is hard work. Getting older I knew I was going to be more susceptible to diseases such as diabetes so that was a motivator, (going away from illness). The way my weight was increasing I could have been in a wheelchair within a few years, but it was also important to visualise myself succeeding (moving towards something). I was driven by the desire to look better and the thought of being able to go into shops and choose clothes I wanted rather than what I could fit in.

Imagining the future

Professional athletes visualise winning a gold medal and the race. They don't just think it would be nice to win it but instead they use all their senses. They visualise, they can see themselves on the podium, they hear the roar of the crowd, they feel the tingling sensation knowing they are a winner, they can taste success...

Imagery can help to enhance our motivation and increase our confidence. We can imagine ourselves working out, exercising, eating healthy food etc.

I've used this technique right from the beginning. In my mind I could see myself as a slim person. I acted like a fit and healthy person. I knew a healthy person would walk briskly, eat slowly, exercise more and demonstrate restraint over goodies so that's what I did most of the time. I spent far more time on this then on visualising the negatives - of me being so fat that I'd never be able to walk, with a fatty liver wearing huge kaftans and with sweat rashes under my boobs and belly.

If you find it hard to visualise then what you might prefer to do is to list all the good things you will gain from losing weight, and also list the reasons for not losing weight. Which list looks more appealing?

Self talk

Whether or not we succeed with weight loss often boils down to what goes on in our heads, the inner self talk. We need to believe that we can succeed, and motivate ourselves with our thoughts. Our self talk can be either positive or negative. Negative self talk is more likely to lead to negative results, and positive self talk leads to positive results and can increase our self confidence. Too often we fill our heads with statements like 'I'll never lose weight'. Our mind then looks for lots of reasons to make this true. If we keep telling ourselves that we can't lose weight, we won't! It's far better to say things such as *'I can lose weight easily, I'm enjoying eating healthy'*. We need to focus more on positive self talk such as *'Each day I'm more healthy'*, or *"I can lose this weight and enjoy the process'*.

We can't be 100% positive, so whenever a negative thought comes into our mind we need to stop the thought from taking over. I find it helpful to both visualise and say out loud the word Stop! I see it as a red stop sign and if I'm alone will say it out loud, or in my head when I'm with others.

Our beliefs can affect our weight

We need to have the inner belief that we can make a change and achieve our desired goal. If we expect to fail we are creating a negative self fulfilling prophecy. This can lead to our actual failure which lowers our self confidence further.

Our beliefs can have a significant impact on weight loss. For example in a clinical trial, patients were given a harmless injection of saline solution but were told it will lead to hair loss. This actually happened to about 35% of the trial sample. Our mind is that powerful.

> **If we believe we can make the changes that will make us more healthy then we will.**

Determination/Self efficacy

We must believe we can be successful if we want to achieve our goals. This determination keeps us going even when the scales haven't dropped. It keeps us focused knowing that if we put the effort in we will get there eventually and this keeps us going through the plateaus, which are normal. This determination also allows us to rebound from failures and set backs with ease.

Have a role model

I didn't want to be a size zero, and I know many slim people are 'skinny fat'. They may be a size 10 but they aren't fit and they eat too many processed foods. My objective was to be strong and healthy. To be able to walk up hills without getting out of breath and not to struggle getting out of a chair. I watched Shakira's video for She-Wolf and loved her dancer's body, with strong legs. Clearly I'm 20 years older than her but I used her as my role model. I had a picture of her in the kitchen, at my desk, and on my phone. I continually asked myself *'What would Shakira do?'* That would be to say no to the cake and yes to any extra 10 minutes on the cross trainer, I imagined!

'If you want to be successful, find someone who has achieved the results you want and copy what they do and you'll achieve the same results'

Tony Robbins

WEEK 1

Saturday, 3 October 2009
Weight: 18 stone 13lb

Ok, so 18 stone 13lbs is not 19 stone, not quite! But, to look at things another way, in a few months time I'm likely to hit 20 stone. Things have got to change, I can't carry on gaining weight or I will cross that line. The last time I weighed myself I was at 18 stone 6lb, this was far too much but I still carried on eating – that's what happens, you get into a pattern and mine involved working hard and then rewarding myself with good food, nice wine and mars bar choc ices.

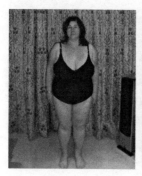 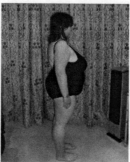 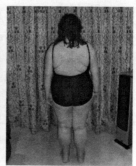

I could waste energy thinking about what I've done and beating myself up but what's the point in that? It won't change the past. What I can do is create a new future.

I'm going to take massive action and I'm going to do things differently. I'm going to stop treating food as my drug of choice to deal with pain - stress, depression, anxiety, over work ... in the past I've calmed myself down with food, given myself a treat with food, and it hasn't made me happier, just fatter! I lie. While I ate, it did make me feel good, but later I felt revulsion and guilt. Not good feelings to have.

Why do I associate writing with eating? Writing is a big part of my work and in the past year I've written three books in eight months. Remember how you revised with a packet of biscuits next to you? That was me with my writing, eating while I thought, eating while I typed and then drinking wine at night after the writing was done.

IT WILL TAKE TIME

It's taken time to put on weight and it will take time to lose it. Too often we want the weight to drop off quickly but that will mean losing muscle and when we lose weight quickly we also regain quickly. If we think in terms of calories, to lose 1 pound a week we need to reduce our weekly calorie intake by 3,500 which equates to 500 less calories a day. It's not quite this simple but these figures do indicate how long it can take.

If you do the maths, being 3 stone overweight means you have taken in 147,000 calories more than you need. You could easily put this on in a year by taking in 400 extra calories a day - which is less than a 100 gram chocolate bar. Over 3 years, this is just 134 calories a day.

I talk to my career coaching clients about having clear outcomes and getting focused, so that's what I'm doing now. I also discuss being accountable. My clients share their goals with me as their coach. This time I'm going to do something very different to what I usually do, which is to go on a diet and not tell anyone. I could then go off it a week later and no one would know. This time I'm going to tell everyone and publically refer to it on my blog, my Facebook page and in my monthly business newsletter.

From today I am going to change my eating habits. I'm quite embarrassed to share this with you but part of my new future is being truthful about what I eat and why. This really was a typical day:

- **Breakfast**: scrambled eggs on buttered toast. My husband makes amazing scrambled eggs, with a big knob of butter.

- **Midmorning**: a few biscuits, or even a couple of chocolate covered club bars.

- **Lunch**: cheese and pickle sandwich and a mars bar ice cream.

- **Mid afternoon**: some fruit, and also some chocolate limes or éclairs.

- **Dinner**: jacket potato, pork chop, lots of vegetables followed by cake and half a bottle of wine.

- **Supper**: cheese and biscuits or a couple of slices of buttered toast.

Some days I'd eat less, but my food intake was getting bigger, as my body was getting used to bigger and bigger meals.

I knew how to eat more healthily so a typical menu for my first week was:

- **Breakfast**: porridge.

- **Lunch**: smoked mackerel, salad and 1 slice of wholemeal bread with a thin coating of butter.

- **Mid afternoon**: apple and banana.

- **Dinner**: Chicken with lots of vegetables and half a jacket potato followed by a yoghurt.

- **Supper**: an apple

- No alcohol!

I also got back into walking and started to wear my pedometer again.

THE BENEFITS OF WALKING

At my heaviest I started exercising with a brisk walk, walking for 15 minutes then walking back, (that was tough enough to start!) gradually increasing the length of time I spent walking. I made it a habit, I would wake up and go straight out, and within a few weeks I was doing a 3 mile walk. It's not just about a 1 hour walk though, it's also about putting more steps into a day and logging progress. I bought a *Fitbug*, to monitor my steps each day, and to see results over time online. I focused on increasing my steps to 10,000 a day and later to 15,000. I was also able to monitor my nutrition and other activity as well.

Monday, 5 October 2009

At this point I know I need to exercise more and walking isn't going to be enough. To give myself a real kick start I decided I'd invest some money in personal training sessions. They can be expensive but when I compared the cost to the cost of going out for meals a couple of nights a week plus buying alcohol and chocolate I think things would probably balance out.

I did my research and found Ben Carpenter. He had a very detailed website with some very useful articles on healthy eating and reaching goals, so I liked what I read. The question was, would he want to work with someone like me? Many trainers want to work with fit and attractive clients, so would a fat 50 something be outside his ideal client profile? I am motivated and I have set goals so that has to count for something.

We exchanged a few emails and arranged to have an introductory meeting on Wednesday. Ben later told me that he is most interested in motivated people and I am certainly that. I decided I would work with him twice a week until Christmas and then move to once a week. Later Ben told me how impressed he was that I had all his articles printed and in a folder and had obviously read them.

Friday, 9 October 2009

Bust	136.5 cm
Biceps, right	36 cm
Waist	133 cm
Hips	138.5 cm
Thigh, right	71.5 cm
Calf, right	50.5 cm

My first session with Ben was not in the gym but in the office. He took 12 measurements with calipers and a tape measure and we discussed what I was eating. I don't think most trainers use calipers but Ben trained with Charles Poliquin who is very hot on measuring subcutaneous fat. The measurements showed me to be very insulin resistant and Ben said that I must eliminate starches - e.g. porridge, bread, pasta, rice, potatoes.

WHEAT AND GLUTEN

Modern wheat can be indigestible due to modern processing methods. It is better to swap it for rye, corn, quinoa, millet or wheat free products. Avoiding grain can lead to weight loss as it stabilizes leptin. Leptin is a hormone that tells our body to reduce hunger and increase fat burning. When we become leptin resistant our body remains hungry and stores more fat.

Ben said a diet high in sugar and grain leads to our body becoming sensitised to insulin and we require more to get the job done. Eating too many grains is the main cause of abnormal insulin levels. One of my symptoms was low blood sugar, feeling dizzy and faint if I didn't eat. It can also have contributed to my depression. Ben said that I should get a blood insulin test, my level needs to be below 3. He also said that my blood pressure should be 120/80 without medication and the ratio of triglyceride /HDL should be below 2.

My previous diet was dire, my current diet was much better, but Ben made some suggestions for improvement – swap the porridge for a protein breakfast and cut out bread/potatoes etc. This would help to reduce my level of insulin resistance and makes it easier to burn fat and lose weight. He also suggested I took fish oil supplements, again to help me to burn fat. My new typical daily plan was:

- **Breakfast**: scrambled eggs and poached mushrooms (no butter).

- **Mid morning**: handful of almonds.

- **Lunch**: smoked mackerel fillet with a huge plate of salad.

- **Mid afternoon**: handful of almonds.

- **Dinner**: chicken and a big plate of vegetables.

- **Evening**: fruit and yoghurt.

INSULIN RESISTANCE

Many people, like me, are unable to process carbohydrate sugars and starches efficiently. After consuming a diet consistently high in sugar and grains, over time our bodies can become desensitized to insulin. We become insulin resistant before succumbing to diabetes. Eating refined carbs which includes fizzy drinks and fruit juice alongside white bread, potatoes, cake and biscuits results in elevated insulin levels and accumulating fat in our fat tissue. The more insulin we secrete, the more likely that our cells and tissues will become resistant to that insulin and the fatter we will get. When we eat a lot of sugar our adrenal glands have to work hard to maintain balance, that's why sweet stuff can make us feel jittery. Even thinking of food can make us secrete insulin so regular eating stops us worrying we won't get enough food. Once we are no longer insulin resistant we can introduce wholemeal bread and brown rice but should still not eat these foods to excess.

I was also to have protein with each meal because I would burn more fat by eating protein. Ben said that my cravings were due to fluctuations in my blood sugar level and I had to eat every 3 hours. He also wanted to test out what I could and couldn't do so I had to show him how far I could squat, this would allow him to prepare for our sessions next week. I'm feeling a little apprehensive but excited too!

DISCLAIMER - This has worked for me, but do check with your doctor before making any changes.

Full details on the way I ate can be found in the appendix of this book. I followed the paleo diet. This diet was based on the following principles:

The Principles

- **Eat clean**: this means avoiding all food that can put stress on the body - alcohol, sugar, coffee, tea, fizzy drinks, chemical additives like aspartame and food colouring. Also dairy, wheat and gluten.

- **Eat protein with every meal**: it stabilises blood sugar, prevents hunger and fuels our muscles.

- **Eat real food**: not processed food, not diet food. If the packaging contains ingredients you haven't heard of, avoid them.

- **Eat enough food**: if you go on a low calorie diet you may lose weight quickly but this is not necessarily fat and could well be muscle.

- **Drink water**: drink 1 litre of water for every 50lbs of body weight. This helps to rid our body of toxins.

- **Drink green tea, and tulsi tea**: these are low or free of caffeine. Green tea can boost your metabolism.

- **Don't count calories**: not all calories were created equally. You could eat a handful of nuts or a chocolate bar. One has vitamins, minerals and good fats, the other contains few nutrients.

You can eat

There are masses of foods you can eat - most meat, fish, vegetables, nuts and seeds are okay. Limited, low fructose fruits like berries and apples are fine too as are healthy fats. The full list can be found in the appendix.

HEALTHY FATS ARE GOOD

Fats get bad press, but fats are not to blame, sugar is! Healthy fats contain Omega 3 essential fatty acids and are found in fish, salmon, walnuts, flax seeds, organic eggs.

You can't eat

Sugar and artificial sweeteners, dairy (not even milk), processed foods with ingredients that weren't available a hundred or more years ago (including diet foods and fizzy drinks), wheat, potatoes, coffee, alcohol, dried fruit, hydrogenated margarine and processed oils.

I was told that the quantities were not important but always to sit down to eat. Also to eat 6 or 7 times a day and never go for more than 3 hours before eating again. The diet isn't a vegetarian diet per se but can probably be adapted. All food to be cooked conventionally, not microwaved.

EATING 7 MEALS A DAY

Our body needs to be fuelled regularly, we then get a sustained release of energy throughout the day and don't get the late afternoon energy drop. The 7 meals in question are not large but instead sufficient food is divided into smaller meals eaten more often.

- **Eat regularly**: eat every 3 hours, don't wait until you are hungry. Your body will appreciate getting regular fuel.

- **Eat slowly and sit down to eat**: so you appreciate the food and also to aid digestion. This is mindful eating. If I want something I need to savour every mouthful, and must put food on a plate, e.g. I shouldn't eat ice cream out of a tub.

- **Get moving**: introduce activity into each and every day.

- **Lift weights**: lifting weights will help build muscle and burn more fat.

- **Don't stress**: being stressed raises cortisol levels and makes our body retain fat around our middle.

- **Log food and times**: measurement makes it easier to notice changes and chart progress.

A weeks food diary

I've included what I ate on various dates through this book. You can also read a weeks food diary in the appendix.

MINDFUL EATING

We multi task. We don't think about what we need to eat or how to eat. We read the paper as we eat breakfast, check emails as we sit in a meeting, eat dinner in front of the TV, eat lunch on the go as we dash across town. All of this leads to mindless eating and fat gain. We should follow the Buddhist concept of mindfulness, paying attention to the colour, smell, texture and flavour of our food and chewing slowly.

When shopping we need to be mindful of food that will enrich our health and don't buy high fat, carb loaded processed foods.

We need to eat in a positive and calm state. When we are stressed our bodies are ready to fight or flee (the stress response) and to enable us to do this blood is diverted from our vital organs, which include the digestive system. Our ability to absorb nutrients drops and we don't feel as satisfied by our food. Due to the anticipated stressful situation our body starts to produce cortisol. This has been linked to weight gain especially around our middle. Eating quickly can be enough to trigger this stress response.

Eat slowly and silently for the first 5 minutes to focus on the food. It takes 20 minutes for our brains to register that we are full and when we rush our food we haven't had a chance to realise that we are full. When we slow down and focus on enjoying our food we will get the full benefit from our food.

It's also about deciding in advance whether we really need to eat that bar of chocolate or bag of crisps. We might prefer a hug! Being mindful also helps to identify when we have had enough and stops us gorging until we are stuffed.

WEEK 2

Monday, 12th October 2009
Weight: 18 stone 7lb
6lb total loss

I already was a member at the gym, but like so many others I just did the same old thing each time I visited. My typical visit involved a 25 minute brisk walk on the treadmill, 20 minutes rowing and then some weights, but I had never increased the difficulty of my regime; I just did the same thing each time. Ben created a programme that we would work through together but I'd also be able to do on my own. My very first programme consisted of:

- **Set A**: 15 step ups on to a step used in step aerobics classes, dumb bell row and dumb bell push.

- **Set B**: a minute on the treadmill, rope face pulls and single leg lowering.

> If you are going to go to the gym an instructor or personal trainer will carefully explain what it is you need to do and probably give you pictures of the exercises too.

Ben strongly believes in writing things down so you can monitor progress. I agree, how can you tell if you are improving if you don't keep track of where you are and where you have come from? It's not just about doing the same things, it is about progression and improvement. So, if I can do 8 reps today, next time I have to do 10 and so on. You can see a couple of example programmes in the appendix.

SET REALISTIC GOALS

Many people want to lose a stone in a month or 10lb in the 2 weeks before a holiday. They follow a highly restricted diet and may lose the weight but this includes water and also muscle, not good! I knew to lose a huge amount of weight I needed to be realistic and set manageable and achievable goals. These were not just about weight loss but also about losing inches, being more flexible, having greater strength and feeling great. I wanted to feel fantastic. Being fit and healthy was my main objective and I love the way I can now walk up all the stairs at a tube station rather than stand in line on an escalator.

When we work towards a goal we feel more positive, motivated and in control of our lives. To be successful our goal must be congruent with our belief system. We have to believe we can achieve it and we need to believe we can be successful. It helps to write the goal down and keep it some place visible. *'I choose to eat foods that will make me healthy and vital'*. I wrote this down and kept it in my car, by my desk, in my handbag and on my bathroom mirror so I could read it regularly.

I was clear about **all** the benefits of achieving this goal - to have more energy, to look better, to feel great, to drop several dress sizes and wear nice clothes. I also considered the obstacles that could get in the way of achieving my goal, in my case the main one being eating whilst travelling with work, and then I created a plan to deal with this.

WEEK 3

Monday, 19th October, 2009
Weight: 18 stone 3lb
10lb total loss

It's been a busy week with no time to write this diary, but I have been logging my food. This past week I went to the gym on my own on Tuesday, with Ben on Thursday and again on my own on Saturday. What I really hate about the gym are the huge mirrors. I don't want to look at me, but I found a place to stand where a pillar obstructed the view of the mirror and felt much better. I still wonder what other people think of this big fat lump. Gyms are full of fit people and the occasional lump like me, but I think I'm the fattest at my gym. Some of these may once have been overweight but many have no idea what it's like to struggle. Just getting through the door is hard, and I want to be invisible. I know why people prefer to exercise at home, that's why I used to go walking, as I felt less embarrassed about my size, but I know I need to use professional equipment and following a work out video wouldn't have been enough. Perhaps a local leisure centre would have been less off putting, but I needed to go to this gym to meet my personal trainer and I need to continue to get through this embarrassment.

MULTIVITAMINS

Ben advised me to take high quality multivitamins to help minimise deficiencies which can stop us losing body fat. Fat loss is essentially nothing more than a large scale detox of the body, the more efficiently we can detox our body the faster we will lose weight as our body becomes more efficient.

Thursday, 22 October 2009

Another busy week, sometimes my consultancy takes me to London and other times I need to focus on writing. I've also been quite stressed. I had a mammogram two weeks ago and they wanted me to attend for further tests. I tried to keep this at the back of my mind and only Simon knew. Normally I would have dealt with emotional stress through food and drink but this time I kept focused on eating healthy and exercising. I knew if I told others they would have worried, and why worry them unnecessarily? It's hard to express how relieved I was to get the all clear. The doctor told me I needed to lose weight and when I described my new found zest for health she was very impressed!

I listen carefully to what Ben tells me and he is clear I have to give up diet cola. But I like it and used to drink 3 or 4 cans in the afternoon. On reflection I think it has been the caffeine boost I crave as I drink these more in the afternoon. He told me that diet cola might be low in calories but it has lots of nasty health implications.

THE DANGER OF LOW CAL DRINKS

We can think low cal drinks are the answer, but they contain artificial sugar which primes our bodies to expect sugar. When we don't get any we experience carb and chocolate cravings. Far better to have 1 glass of non diet fizzy drink if we must.

Drinks that sound healthy can be just as bad. I thought Vitamin Water would be a better choice, but each 500ml bottle contains 26g of sugar so clearly not.

I have been 100% committed to my new eating plan with no deviation at all. I think previously I've thought it okay to have a little extra here and there – a glass of wine or two, a couple of cheese and biscuits, some chocolate biscuits … and before long I've forgotten I'm on my diet.

FAD DIETS WORK IN THE SHORT TERM

Fad diets like the Maple Syrup diet or the Baby Food diet will work in the short term because they are boring or unpleasant but as soon as we stop following them the weight goes back on.

So I'm following my eating plan and following my exercise plan. Ben has set me on a series of exercises and he has one rule – each time you have to go that little bit further – so if I have done 12 repetitions last time, it need to do 14 repetitions next time. I'm working out with him twice a week and last week also went to the gym on my own 3 times. I'm also now taking fish oil after each meal.

FISH OIL

Fish oil is an excellent source of Omega 3 fatty acids. Charles Poliquin says that fish oil is the most important supplement to get depressed people off their duff and into the gym. Many people take 1 tab of cod liver oil a day but that won't make a difference.

Due to my huge size I needed to take it in liquid form, I'd be on about 18 tablets with each meal otherwise. I take Eskimo 3 stable fish oil which comes from the oily fish living in the deep seas of the Antarctic and South Atlantic, and is of a higher quality than cod liver oil. This mitigates the insulin response, which means it helps with weight loss and is taken after each meal.

I started on 30ml a day, which is a 5ml spoon 6 times a day. By 16th February I was able to drop to 20ml a day.

I already have a lot more energy and it's great to try on trousers that were a snug fit last time to find that they are now loose. In just 2 weeks my fitness has also increased. With my current exercise programme, I have made great progress: Ben made me do step ups holding a 3kg weight in each hand, I couldn't believe how hard it was to start with and wanted to stop before the target of 15 but he was very motivational, kept telling me not to give up, I could do it and I did! The dumbbell row is now done with a weight increase from 8kg to 10kg and I now do the dumbbell push with 8kg instead of 7kg. My strength is improving on all fronts. On the treadmill I'm only jogging for 1 minute but to me it feels like 20. The first time I only managed it twice at 7.2kph but now I'm up to doing it 4 times at 8.0kph. I now do rope pulls on the 30kg setting instead of the 20kg setting and I can do 26 repetitions of the single leg lowering whereas before I could only do 12!

GOAL SETTING

Setting goals focuses our attention and helps keep us persistent. When I discuss goal setting with my career coaching clients we discuss goals being **SMARTER**.

We need a goal which is **Specific**. We are clear on about what we want to achieve. It needs to be **Measurable**, we need to know where we start from (weight, what the tape measure says, how we feel) so we can monitor progress. The goal has to be **Achievable** - we can achieve a % weight loss but it might be unrealistic to weigh 9 stone. It also has to be **Realistic** - losing weight is achievable, changing our height is not. My realism meant that I planned to lose weight slowly, I was in this for the long term.

Time bound means we have a time scale to achieve. We may not know specifically how long it can take and the final stone or so can take a long time to lose, but we can focus on eating healthy and exercising more for 3-6 months and then review progress. The goal should also be **Exciting**, it should have personal meaning for us, it has to be something that we want to do. Finally it should be **Recorded**. We need to write it down and monitor progress, just like I have done.

Our goals can include both the long term goal, for me it was to lose over 10 stone in weight in total, but also shorter goals, e.g. to visit the gym 4 times a week, to walk 10,000 steps a day, to eat clean for a week.

We also need to be aware of possible setbacks, my sports injury and medical treatment meant that I needed to adjust my goals.

WEEK 4

Monday, 26th October 2009
Weight: 18 stone 0 lb
13lb total loss

On Friday Ben changed my programme. I understand why personal trainers do this, and why we need to, because our body needs to be shocked into change. It was challenging but I worked as hard as I could and really concentrated on my breathing which helped.

THE GYM DOES NOT EQUAL A CHOCOLATE BAR

If we work really hard at the gym we can use up about 500

[text obscured]

faster [text obscured] not so much the smell and taste but the [text obscured] my throat, and I'm having to take it 6 times a [text obscured] Remember, I'm eating 6 small meals a day.

My cloth[es are] getting so loose on me that I'll need to buy more. I'm going to buy low cost clothes, and buy them tight as an incentive to get into them. Last week I bought some trousers that I could barely zip up, these went up much easier today. I also checked on some other trousers. When I started my black linen ones had a gap of four fingers across my tummy so I was a long way off doing them up, but they are almost okay now. Such a great feeling, it shows that what I'm doing is working. I'm more used to the horror and shame of realising that I can no longer fit into clothes. No wonder I'd moved into stretchy clothes.

THE PERILS OF STRETCH CLOTHING

Fat people wear clothes with stretch. They feel more comfortable but this also means we don't notice when we are putting on weight. I'd convince myself I was only a size 28 in my stretch tops and trousers even though I had to wear a size 32 with clothes that fitted, like jeans. Never again did I buy clothes without lycra and the first thing I did was cut the labels out of them.

Thursday, 29 October 2009

I'd never intended to go to the gym on Tuesday, too busy with work. I also knew going on Wednesday would be difficult, I'd have had to leave the house by 7am and now that it's Autumn I'm not waking up until 7am so I didn't go. But I also didn't feel well, beginning to get a sore throat and not feeling 100%, I even noticed a spot!

I did get some exercise though. On Tuesday night we saw Ash at Gloucester Guildhall and I'm back on form with enough energy and stamina to stand all night and dance! Burn, baby burn! (That's one of their songs!)

Thursday I had another session with Ben, I told him I wasn't feeling 100% and it was a very hard day. Usually I find Ben's push to do more repetitions each time highly motivating but today it was a bit annoying, I wanted to do less. I was really sweating so this must be doing me good, but gosh it was hard and my legs were wobbly after just one set. I did try to rest more between sets this time, but Ben wouldn't let me sit for too long, he kept pushing me forward. I'm doing four reps of the first set and Ben gave me an option of dropping to three today, but I stuck with the four. I think I would have felt that I'd let myself down if I had taken the easier option. This was such a hard work out, but it was very satisfying to have done it.

Friday, 30 October 2009

I'm now on Dr Mercola's mailing list and today watched one of his videos on the importance of high quality protein for breakfast. He said that most people approach breakfast and lunch and 'fail to plan and plan to fail', accordingly making poor breakfast food choices. We need to plan what we will eat, especially if we are going to be travelling.

EATING FAT DOES NOT MAKE US FAT. EXCESS CARBOHYDRATES IN OUR DIET MAKES US FAT

Wholemeal bread and cereal are fine to eat, but not in unlimited quantities, and when you are as fat as me these carbs will lead to fat storage. I can introduce these when weight is within healthy limits.

my 20s and to the 16 stone mark around my 50th birthday. I still have another 2 stone to lose to get me back there, whereas I could be slim by now if I'd kept my focus.

DIETS CAN MAKE US FAT

Research has found that most people who go on a diet end up being more over weight as they have messed up their metabolism through starvation. The great benefit of my approach is my body gets all the nutrients it needs and I am more healthy than I've ever been.

I've now completed 3 weeks with Ben and today we had a second measurement day, again with both the tape measure and calipers. Three weeks ago Ben wasn't able to take all the caliper readings as my body was too dense in places. He managed to measure more areas this time which is good, and I think this means that my fat is turning to muscle or at least beginning to break down. Based on the measurements he took I've dropped by 15.5mm overall in 3 weeks. It might not sound much but this is good! Tape measurements make more sense to most and you can see below how I've shaved 2 inches off my waist already.

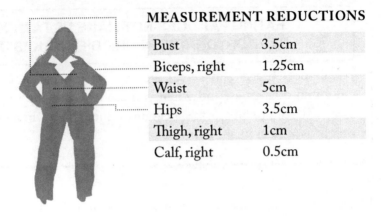

MEASUREMENT REDUCTIONS

Bust	3.5cm
Biceps, right	1.25cm
Waist	5cm
Hips	3.5cm
Thigh, right	1cm
Calf, right	0.5cm

CARB CYCLING

Ben introduced me to carb cycling to enhance weight loss. For 14 days I eat 'clean', this includes everything listed in the appendix under the Paleo diet except fruit. On day 15 I can eat 'treat food' after each meal – it's not a day to go mad. I have to eat my meal first but can follow this with a treat. E.g. porridge or cereal for breakfast, for lunch bread or pasta, and dinner could be cake after my main meal.

I was apprehensive. How will it affect me? Will I enjoy it or will I be scared that it will set me off again on cravings?

Ben said said that what's more likely to happen is that I will feel ill afterwards. After this special day I then eat 'clean' for 5 days, but on the fifth day I can have carbs after my evening meal. And so on. This enhances fat loss.

I think the reason for this is that at the moment I'm avoiding processed carbs, and if I continue this for an extended period of time the glycogen in my muscles will drop so my body will burn muscle not fat and I don't want that.

As Ben had spent 30 minutes on measurements there was no time for my usual weight training. Instead I rode on the bike as fast as I could for 40 seconds, on level 11 then a slower pace for 80 seconds and continued for 20 minutes. This was very hard going, but working at a high intensity then slowing down until I recover and then starting again is a great way to burn fat.

Saturday, 31 October 2009

When you have a busy job it can be hard to find the time to get to the gym, especially at the weekend when I spend more time with Simon. This morning we went shopping but I put more exercise into my day, I ran up the stairs at the department store and ran up the stairs at WH Smiths twice.

Ben suggested I start taking Psyllium husks. I have to put a spoonful in a glass of water and to drink it after each meal. This is to rid my body of 'waste' and thus lose more fat. It is partly to fill me up but also slows down the absorption of sugar into my blood stream, so it's a very healthy thing to do even if it seems weird.

PSYLLIUM HUSK

Psyllium comes from the seed of the Plantago Ovato plant and is an excellent source of soluble dietary fibre. This acts like a sponge, absorbing waste material in the bowels. Ben said to take a spoonful in a glass of water and to drink it after each meal. This would rid my body of 'waste' and thus I would lose more fat. It can turn to the consistency of wallpaper paste, so I found the best way to take it is to put water in a shaker, add a spoonful and drink it back as fast as possible so it swells up inside me, not in the container. Rinse the glass or container well or the husks stick to the sides and you can't get them off.

I decided not to take the psyllium husks this morning – just in case I had a sudden urge to go to the loo while out shopping, but for lunch and my evening meal I followed each meal with a rounded 5ml spoon. I'm off to a conference on Wednesday, will I stick to my eating plan? I wonder how will I manage, especially with the carb cycling, but if I plan everything it should be fine.

'It takes as much energy to wish as it does to plan.'

Sunday, 1 November 2009

I've only lost 0.5lbs this week? Why? It really is a bit disappointing. Even though Ben has said that it's inches which are important - especially those around my middle - I know I'm making healthy food choices and I've done 4 hours in the gym this week so it just doesn't seem fair.

Working out properly at the gym is new to me. In the past I would have just continued to do the same thing again and again, never really pushing myself. Now I have much more focus.

Today I got to the gym at about 9am. I decided to work really hard, and did, increasing the repetitions for each exercise from Thursday.

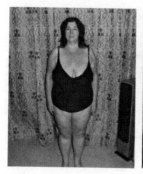 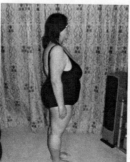 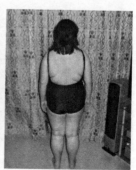

One of the exercises I do is to lift weights from a lying position on a bench. All goes well until it's time to get off the bench. It's really hard to do with my crap stomach muscles. When I work out with Ben he helps me to get up but doing it on my own has been hard. I've had to roll off the bench - not pretty - but today I managed to sit up myself. That's quite an achievement and it's one of the little things I've noticed which illustrates my overall improvement.

As planned, I had my protein shake immediately after my workout but this time still felt a bit light headed after my shower. Was this because I'd pushed myself hard or was it because I hadn't eaten anything since 8.30pm last night? I didn't eat till 11am today as I failed to allow enough time to eat before leaving for the gym.

Despite the fact I'm going to a conference next week I decided to start the carb cycling and will contact the hotel to organise a special diet which shouldn't be too difficult - protein and salad.

I think the psyllium husks are taking effect, I'm pooing more and I think this is because it's clearing out my bowels (sorry if I am giving you an image here), but I also remember reading that it can swell to 20 times its size in your tummy, like a big sponge. Certainly today I've felt a lot less hungry and I had to make myself eat. Just realised I haven't had a snack mid morning or afternoon – suppose I need to munch on veggies, so I decided to split my evening meal in two.

I just don't feel hungry at all so hope this will lead to a significant drop this week.

LOW CARB MEALS

Low carb meals mean we can feel satisfied without calorie counting. We aren't excluding carbs, we'll still get these from vegetables.

WEEK 5

Monday, 2 November 2009
Weight: 17 stone 13.5lbs
13.5lbs total loss

I'm enjoying going to the gym. This was my first time going through the

warned against doing an exercise incorrectly (it wouldn't be doing much
good) so I thought it best to book another session to make sure I've got
things right. I'm now focused. I know what I'm going to do. Previously, I
would really just mooch about, feeling I'd done a good job simply because
I showed up. I never had the focus I now have. I like having a programme
to follow and I like the way I monitor my progress.

CONSISTENCY

We can't go to the gym a couple of times and think that this
will be enough. It takes time to make a change and a plan
keeps us on the right track.

Luckily Ben could fit me in on Monday and we did considerably more.
I felt absolutely exhausted at the end of the session, almost felt like I
was going to collapse. He said it had to do with depleting my protein
stores. He advised me to buy some protein powder and to take some
straight after my workout. In retrospect, I should have had my protein
powder with me or to have eaten some protein when I got home, but
the exhaustion took over and I literally collapsed on my chair. I usually
keep going; this is the first time I've found I can't. Not actually sure it
is doing me good to feel like this.

PROTEIN SHAKES

Protein shakes ensure I don't lose muscle after my weights sessions at the gym. I use an unflavoured whey protein powder which does not contain sucrolose or sugar. I add cinnamon for taste and this also helps to burn more fat.

WHEY PROTEIN POWDER

To build muscle we must eat enough protein, taking whey protein powder after a workout means that the weight I lose will be fat not muscle and helps encourage my body to repair itself.

WHAT TO WEAR AT THE GYM

It's tempting to put on a huge baggy t-shirt and old sweat pants but I found if I looked the best I could it gave me more confidence. I didn't buy tight lycra but a V neck t-shirt made my bust look better than a round necked t-shirt and some jogging pants that fitted me created a good look. None of my clothes were expensive, I was going down the sizes quite rapidly, but they did help me feel better about myself. I also invested in a sports bra - essential to stop my boobs going all over the place.

The worst part of going to the gym is having to shower; a normal towel doesn't cover me and even the bigger bath sheet I use doesn't meet leaving a gap exposing so much wobbly flesh.

My second day of carb cycling and my appetite has dropped. When I later talked about this with Ben he said that when we eat food which isn't very nutritious our body craves more food to get what it wants. Now I'm eating such high quality food my body is getting all it needs. I must continue to eat this way!

I continue to drink lots of water. Drinking a litre for every 50 pounds of body weight means that at almost 18 stone I need to drink 5 litres (nearly 9 pints) and this is in addition to the water I drink at the gym. I have to keep a tally in my diary to make sure I do this. As I lose weight I can cut back on the water.

It's been a very hard session with Ben at the gym today. He keeps moving me forward and I can now do 34 squats with a gym ball behind my back. I do 4 exercises in set A and 3 exercises in set B. I've now progressed so that I can do the squats holding 6kg in each hand.

Some of the increases in weight astound me, I would never have believed I could have made such great progress. I've been doing the 'Bent over dumbbell row' with 10kg weights. This time I had to move up to 15kg (the 10s were too easy, the 12s were broken and someone was using the 14kg ones. I only managed to lift them 6 times but was still very pleased, I would have thought this was impossible! Throughout this session I felt pushed to my limit, but that's why I'm paying to work out with Ben.

I'm noticing the other people at the gym. Most do the same thing every time. When you exercise like this you think you are being good, going to the gym 3 times a week, but it's not really doing much. Not like what I've been doing for the past 3 weeks. It's hard to believe that I did my first work out with Ben on the 12th October. 4 weeks of healthy eating but only 3 weeks of serious training at the gym. Life has changed so much!

READY MEALS

Read the packaging and notice there are numerous ingredients that are not natural including a lot of chemicals. These, like sugar, are toxins to the body. Our liver has to work very hard to get rid of these toxins and again this can lead to weight gain as our body is under stress.

I am having cravings. These are good cravings - I want to eat an apple, not a chocolate orange! But for 2 weeks I can't eat fruit at all. In the past I'd normally give in, and it would be easy to do so. I used to think 'well, just one won't hurt' and that was one magnum, not one chocolate finger. But I will not give in – the cravings will pass and I opt for another glass of water. I really am drinking a lot of water.

TO LOSE FAT

I've read masses of books as part of my research including one by Gary Taubes - 'Good Calories, Bad Calories'. He says that to lose fat you need to restrict carbs and keep blood sugar and insulin levels low. Most people think to lose weight you should follow a low cal diet, and the notion that carbs make us fat goes against what most people think, but it works. We also need to eat regularly to keep levels stable.

WEEK 6

Monday, 9 November 2009
Weight: 17 stone 9lbs
18lbs total loss

Last week I weighed 17 stone 13.5lbs and I felt so disappointed. This past week I've been even stricter – cutting fruit out for 2 weeks and taking psyllium husk. It's been a slightly unusual week because I was at a conference for 3 days and was unable to get to the gym. A gym session consumes not only the time spent in the gym, but also the time needed to make my hair look good afterwards.

THE NEED TO PLAN

I planned for the conference. It's easy to go with the moment and get distracted from your goals. Not this time. I'd arranged for a special diet and even got to talk with the executive chef on arrival. Wednesday evening I had a salad to start followed by steak and veggies, breakfast the next day was smoked salmon and a boiled egg, lunch was chicken salad, conference dinner was halibut and salad with a salad to start. I was still a bit hungry and as I was seated with people eating and drinking I asked for some nuts for dessert, so that was good! Similar food on Friday. I did as much walking up stairs as I could, actually running up two and three flights of stairs.

I was expecting a decent loss and I've got it; 4.5lbs, yippee! Seeing the difference on the scales really makes me motivated. It's not just the weight loss, it's the fitness. At the conference I won a second National Career Award but didn't celebrate with champagne, I was happy without it.

ORANGE JUICE

Orange juice is full of sugar and as it has no fibre it's far better to eat an orange instead. The reason we drink it is down to good marketing by the Florida orange suppliers.

Last Tuesday Ben changed my workout for the third time. No more doing squats with a ball, I'm now doing them on my own – brilliant! Other exercises have changed too and I am really pushing myself. For example, Ben asked me to use a set of 8kg weights but I couldn't find them so I went for a 9kg set. Yesterday I went on my own, did more than with Ben and as I couldn't find the 9kg set I pushed myself to use the 10s. I loved the fact that the man next to me was using 8s! This week we've introduced rowing as fast as I can – this means I'm burning fat quicker!

Friday, 13 November 2009

Nearly a week since my last diary entry and I'm now recapping the past 5 days. It's been a busy week. 3 days at a conference meant that work backed up and I'm still catching up. In the past when I've been working hard I've 'treated' myself by eating lots of high fat food. I would normally eat almost continuously as I did heavy brain work, but no more – I drink my water, lots of it, and eat regularly. I no longer get the urges to eat sweets and choc ices. I think some of this can be attributed to a change in mindset, I can now see chocolate and not be interested at all. Why would I want to put crap like that in my body?

I had 3 good days in the gym where I worked out, spent the weekend on my own and spent Monday with Ben. I saw Ben again yesterday and I'm now doing my ball squats with 5kg weights in each hand. Yesterday I did 15 of these – amazing when I look back at how few I did at the beginning.

SQUATS
'THE SQUAT IS THE KING OF EXERCISES' PAUL CHEK

I've been reading up on exercises and squatting is one of the best exercises we can do with numerous health benefits including improvements to our digestion and removal of waste. Paul Chek says that it is a primal movement and requires us to use every muscle in our body.

Ben had told me not to work out with weights for more than 3 days in a row. On Tuesday I had planned to do my fast cycling but when I woke up feeling tired, I had to decide whether to do something when I didn't feel I'd give it 100% or to take a rest. I opted for the latter, and I'm glad I did. Sometimes 'going for the burn' and pushing yourself too hard isn't the right thing to do. You can't use this as an excuse regularly but sometimes your body is telling you something and you do need to listen. I had pushed myself hard over the weekend and Ben pushed me further still.

I've continued to make progress on fast rowing but it is very hard – 250 metres rowing as fast as I can. Since the first time I did this, on 3rd November, I am now doing it 4 times instead of 3 and have shaved 7 seconds off my time (70 seconds to 63 seconds on my first set and 5 seconds off the second). I'm also now doing my dumb bell press ups on a ball and have increased from 3 sets using the 9kg weights to 4 sets using the 10kg weights without doing fewer repetitions.

Overall I've been happy with my eating and drinking. I'm on my second week of carb cycling – basically no potatoes, bread etc, nor any fruit. This week I'm taking apple fibre instead of psyllium husk. Ben has said to alternate between one and the other each week so my body doesn't become too accustomed to either. Apple fibre is much nicer! I'm still on the fish oil and will be on it for the rest of my life, but I will reduce the dose as I get slimmer.

APPLE FIBRE

Apple fibre is another good source of soluble fibre. It's got a pleasant apple taste and helps to enhance weight loss as it has a mild appetite suppressing effect. It also helps to stabilise fat levels in our blood stream. It has to be taken with plenty of water so I drink it with 1 pint of water and follow that with another large glass.

The carb cycling ends on Sunday. It's tough but I'm sticking with it. The only day I was less happy with my food was Tuesday. This was the day I felt really tired and I'd run out of salad stuff in the house so ate more protein than veggies. Looking back I don't think that was a good move – a chicken leg for lunch and again for an early tea as we were going out to see Muse in concert. I knew I'd be hungry so I took along a bag of pistachio nuts. I felt I need to compensate over the next couple of days and I cut out my more calorie dense foods.

WEEK 7

Monday, 16 November 2009
Weight: 17 stone 6lbs
21lbs total loss

I was very worried about weighing myself today, thinking that maybe I'd not eaten enough. So it was with trepidation that I got on the scales, but good news, I've lost 3lbs, so now I've lost exactly one and a half stone in 6 weeks. This progress gives me the motivation I need to keep going.

Ben has asked me to take photos so we can monitor my progress. I did but didn't share them with him. It's really hard reviewing them. I don't like looking at photos of me as I don't normally look at myself closely and I look big and fat and horrible. I've joked in the past that I have reverse anorexia, if I'm careful how I stand when I look in a mirror I think I'm fine. I know I need these photos so I can see how things change, but it is still absolutely horrible to look at them. I'm always telling Simon off for taking such rubbish photos, he makes me look fat but if I'm honest I know it's not his technique but me as the subject. Being so fat it is hard to take a flattering photo. I do wear a lot of shawls, I always think these are good at covering up my huge bust.

A new workout today. I'd actually emailed Ben and asked if I could continue with the same one, but no, I had to do a new one. I felt a bit sad to leave that workout behind as I was enjoying it and wanted to carry on and build up on the weights, but Ben doesn't want my body to get used to one programme and he changes it once I've done it 6 times. This time I'm doing revised squats, with my feet elevated at an angle on blocks (the steps from a stepper) and fast rowing for 400m rather than 250m which is tough! My seated row is with heavier weights and my treadmill running has increased by 50%. I've got a new exercise, a seated dumbbell press. I'm also doing push ups on a high step.

Ben advised me not to do weights so regularly as it will be too hard to make gains in strength or endurance, but instead to go for 30 minute sprint sessions in between, so let's see how that goes.

I'm coming to the end of my 2 week carb cycling and I was concerned about what to eat on Sunday. I can eat carbs but which ones? Ben sat down and talked me through what to eat – so the plan is:

- **Breakfast** – follow with porridge
- **Lunch** – roast potatoes
- **Supper** – pineapple

Then back to the strict eating plan for 5 days. I can have carbs after my evening meal on day 5. I think it will be porridge. I have to eat it in one sitting, I can't eat it later. I can also introduce fruit again but just berries.

I'm learning so much from Ben – I asked if tinned tomatoes were okay. He said yes as long as they don't contain sugar. Citric acid is fine. Also, when I start to eat more fruit, thin skinned fruit is good but not yellow fruit such as bananas, melon and pineapple which contain too much sugar. This might sound strict, but I'm finding it easier to have a list of what I can and can't eat rather than to try and limit quantities or count calories. There are masses of things that I can eat and all are listed in the appendix.

WILL POWER

Losing weight can be like quitting smoking or alcohol, but the difference is that we still have to eat every day. Eating 'clean' and planning what to eat enabled me to have a plan to deal with temptation and kept me focused.

Tuesday, 17 November 2009

Yesterday was carbs day – a really odd day, I can eat things I don't normally eat, but I don't want to. Ben had even said that I could eat chocolate but I don't trust myself not to binge on it. He said that I'd feel so bad that it would really put me off, but am I going to take that risk? So for breakfast I had my scrambled eggs and then about two thirds of a standard portion of porridge. For lunch I had chicken and salad followed by some pineapple. For dinner; a proper roast dinner with ribs of beef, lots of veggies and 4 roast potatoes plus a glass of hibiscus juice. I'd bought it as we drank it in Egypt and I knew if I didn't drink it now when would I?

I weighed myself yesterday morning and I'd put on a pound but I know that weight fluctuates. Ben had warned me that I'd put on weight as my glycogen stores took on the carbs so I was surprised this morning to find I was down to 17 stone 5lbs. I want to do everything right and if I'm not sure if something is okay, I must check with Ben.

DON'T KEEP WEIGHING YOURSELF

Our weight fluctuates as we deplete and replete our glycogen stores. For every gram of glycogen, stored or lost, 3gms of water are also stored or lost. I know if I eat carbs my weight will increase by about 3lbs but drop again when I go back to my low carb diet.

I went to the gym yesterday and, building on the work I'd done with Ben on Friday, I felt like I had had a serious workout. Plus, I just went earlier today. As my sessions with Ben are at 4pm I tend to go at that time on my own, but today I have a client from 1pm till 4pm and they could be late so I had a morning session instead. I did 30 minute sprints – they are hard work – going as fast as I could for 40 seconds and then cycling slower until I got my breath back.

Thursday, 19 November 2009

A busy week with work and no time to write my diary but everything is on target. I've stopped keeping my food diary as everything is just as it should be and I'm doing my best to eat my 6 meals a day. Actually, sometimes I've missed out on a mid afternoon meal but with going to the gym I'm having my protein shakes so that is probably okay.

This week I've been to the gym every day – Sunday my programme, Monday sprints, Tuesday my programme and Wednesday sprints. Ben says this is an aggressive policy – it needs to be as I want to have lost 3 stone in 3 months.

I've never worked as hard in my life as I did today. I'm now doing 4 sets of the full programme – in a week I'm now doing elevated squats holding 4kg weights in each hand. My press ups are much smoother and when rowing for 400m I've increased to doing this 4 times instead of 3 and maintained my speed. My dumbbell presses are now done with an extra kg in weight. I've upped my seated rows by 5kg and my treadmill sprints- wow! I've gone from 2 sprints at 7.3kmph to 4 sprints at 7.5kmph.

I wrote earlier about how odd it was to have a carb day and that I'm really scared about letting myself go and losing my focus. Ben said he eats ice cream as his carb food but if I had a litre in the fridge would I be tempted? We also spoke about how I might like to have a drink and how to fit that into my eating plan. What I need to do is to have alcohol as my carbs so I can have champagne on Saturday night!

GET ENOUGH SLEEP

Most of us don't get enough sleep, putting our bodies under stress. Ideally we should sleep for 9-10 hours a day and we should move into the deep sleep pattern roughly 90 minutes after getting into bed. This is when our body diverts blood away from the brain and into our muscles and glands. The adrenal glands in particular are working hard during this time whilst our gall bladder dumps toxins. The earlier we get to sleep the better for muscle recovery and overall physical well being.

NIGHT TIME RITUAL

A night time ritual can include taking Zinc and Magnesium tablets. Magnesium helps to repair lean tissue, helps with insulin sensitivity and cortisol reduction. Insufficient Zinc intake leads to a slow metabolism. I take a combined pill at least 30 minutes before bed to increase the length and quality of my sleep. These should be taken on an empty stomach so I wait an hour from my evening food before taking them. I plan to go to bed before 11pm and as close to 10.30pm as I can. For the hour before bed I don't watch adrenalin pumping TV or check emails and I have a routine which includes a caffeine free drink and a calming book.

Friday, 20 November 2009

I was excited about weighing myself this morning, fully expecting to be 17 stone 03 I'd weighed myself on Wednesday morning and I was 17 stone 04 and a half but now I'm really disappointed. How come the scales are showing me at 17 stone 07, what's going on? I now feel so much fatter, and surely the extra weight can't be muscle? I've worked so hard this week, doing even more than usual. Why did I bother, I'm really annoyed. Okay I came back to this an hour later, I'm actually only 1lb heavier than last week and that could be muscle but why haven't I lost weight? Just checking back and 3 weeks ago I had only lost half a pound but the following week lost 4 and a half so maybe this is going to be similar – I hope so!

LOSING WEIGHT IS NOT A LINEAR PROCESS

Wouldn't it be great if we were like machines and if we could lose weight simply by reducing the amount that we eat? Unfortunately it's not that simple. Our bodies hold water in our glycogen stores. There's a great story of a farmer, he plants seeds and waters the soil but each day when he checks nothing has grown. The farmer doesn't give up, however, he knows results takes time. It's the same with losing weight and getting healthy. Things are happening but this is not always obvious externally so we have to stick at it. As the weeks go by I'm increasing my muscle, I'm getting stronger, I'm becoming more flexible, my metabolic rate is improving, my clothes fit better, I feel more alive.

Met Ben for my session – measurement time. As you can see below I've had some significantly different results so I know I'm losing fat. All of these measurements are from when I started with Ben in October, not from my fattest. 4 cm off my bust and hips!

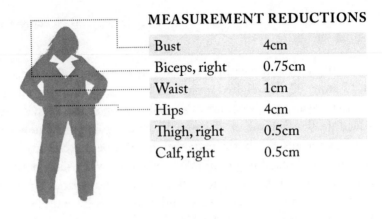

MEASUREMENT REDUCTIONS

Bust	4cm
Biceps, right	0.75cm
Waist	1cm
Hips	4cm
Thigh, right	0.5cm
Calf, right	0.5cm

We also did a revised sprints workout. What I now do is:

Treadmill at 9.1kph for 45 seconds with a 2 minute walk, rower, 200m at level 10, cycle sprints at level 10 for 45 seconds. I did 2 sets with Ben and 2 on my own – he said it was hard and it was!

Saturday, 21 November 2009

Ben suggested I take flaxseed as an alternative to psyllium husk and apple fibre but I don't like it. It doesn't seem anywhere near as good as the psyllium husk or apple fibre for keeping my 'visits' regular!

My mother in law rang this afternoon and offered to take us out for a meal. I said no as I couldn't be certain how the food was cooked so she has offered to cook – I was very clear about what I could and couldn't eat and I think I came across as evangelical but I'm not deviating from my plan for any reason. In the evening we went to see friends and I had one large glass of wine and skipped all the cheese and snacks.

TIP: Stay focused and plan ways to deal with meals out.

Sunday, 22 November 2009

Woke this morning, straight on the scales and I'm 17 stone 06, so I'm back to what I was just over a week ago – I'm feeling so fed up, I thought I'd see a drop on the scales today. Well it is a pound, but that's nothing. Previously I'd just give up if it was like this and eat some high sugar/fat food. It really is hard to resist some nice food and last night I would have really enjoyed eating some cheese but I held back, thinking of the greater good.

TIP: Don't let the scales rule your life, they are only one measure of progress, we also have actual tape measurements and can also think about how much more energy we have.

MEASURES OF SUCCESS

It's not just about what the scales say. It's also about the changes we notice on the tape measure, how we feel and increases in fitness level such as finding it easier to get out of a chair. It's also about those little thing like no longer having to turn sideways when walking down a train aisle and one of my favourites - when the towel finally meets when I wrap myself after a shower.

WEEK 8

Monday, 23 November 2009
Weight: 17 stone 4lbs
23lbs total loss

I've lost 2lbs so that makes me feel much better, and I'd love to shave off another 2lbs by Friday to get me closer to the 2 stone loss overall – still aiming for a minimum of 2.5 stone off by Christmas.

Okay, a new week and it's time to refocus and list not only what I eat but the times I eat. I've set up a food diary for the week and listed when I will eat. I've been making a note of three main meals – breakfast, lunch and dinner and three snacks in between. Ben says I shouldn't be having snacks I should be having six proper meals of smaller size. However, it's hard to always sit down for a proper meal when I have clients here. Maybe I should tell them I need a 10 minute break if they are here for a 3 – 4 hour session. Most clients are aware of my healthy living campaign via my blog and newsletter so I could just be up front with them.

NOT A DIET - HEALTHY EATING

Avoid yo-yo dieting, we will end up fatter in the long run. Success comes from sustainable, healthy changes not temporary ones.

I'm highly focused this week and maybe small differences add up to big changes? Here's my food diary for today, and there are more examples in the appendix.

08.45	Breakfast, 2 scrambled eggs cooked without fat plus multi vits and fish oil.
11.00	1 brazil nut, 12 blueberries, fish oil.
12.00	Lunch, rib eye steak and green beans, fish oil, multi vits and flaxseed in water.
14.15	Protein drink after 30 minutes of sprints
18.00	Chicken and a massive plate of salad
21.30	Chicken, 6 cherry tomatoes and fish oil

Tuesday, 24 November 2009

I've decided to plan even more carefully so I've prepared my midmorning snack so that I can eat it before my 11.00 appointment gets here. I've also put my food diary on my pin board so I can easily write down what I eat.

Wednesday, 25 November 2009

I've never watched *Supersize-Superskinny* before but I did last night. They spoke about Beyonce's diet – maple syrup, cayenne pepper and water (150 calories a day) and someone who lost 7 stone in 6 months eating baked beans – was that it? Obviously this is unhealthy but I can understand why people are tempted by these drastic diets! But how would you do any exercise when you are starving? I also have read through a whole load of material from Dr Mercola's online site. He writes a lot of sense but some things are a bit extreme, I'm already doing a lot of what he says but it threw up a lot of questions.

I'm still logging food carefully and making sure I eat regularly. I'm also thinking about portion size, I'm taking one meal and dividing it into two, so for breakfast I had half a mackerel fillet with tomatoes and had the second half mid morning.

GLYCEMIC INDEX (GI) AND GLYCEMIC LOAD (GL)

The GI scale measures the effects of carbs and sugar on our body. Low GI food releases energy slowly so we feel fuller for longer. High GI food causes elevated levels of insulin. Portion size is also important, we can't eat large quantities just because they are low GI foods.

All low GI food are also low on the Glycemic index, but some foods which are medium or high on the GI scale can have a low GL load. For example, watermelon has a high GI but a relatively low GL.

One of my questions to Ben was on carrots. Dr Mercola says that cooked carrots are high in sugar, should I eat less of these? Ben said that carrots are high on the GI scale but low on the GL scale and are fine to eat.

I decided to check my BMI and it is 40.3, at my heaviest it was 52.4, more than half my weight was fat! I'm still in the morbidly obese category, however.

Thursday, 26 November 2009

I saw the doctor this morning and have organised an insulin fasting test for next week. She said that men are at far greater risk of heart disease than women. I've also signed up for vitamin D testing via a US site. I'm getting even stricter on my food and have given up on drinking milk, which I should have done right from the beginning. Simon does think I'm a bit obsessed but I want to put my health first.

VITAMIN D

This is essential for the absorption of calcium and to maintain strong bones and teeth. It also helps our immune system. Whilst we can get it from the sun, most of us don't get enough so supplements can help. I signed up with Grassroots Health to have my vitamin D levels tested. When I started my level was 13, within 6 months I was up to 29. Six months on I was at 39. The optimal level is 50-65 ng/ml so I'm getting there!

So much of what we read concerning exercise focuses on aerobic exercise such as jogging. This is good for burning calories whilst we're in the gym and for a short time afterwards but we also need to lift weights. This builds muscle, muscle is calorie-hungry and therefore weight lifting increases our metabolic rate helping to burn more fat over time. I was a bit concerned that I'd end up looking like Arnold Schwarzenegger but women don't have enough testosterone in their bodies for this to happen and most men would be only too pleased to have defined muscles.

Yesterday I went back on the psyllium husk. I also started a new programme at the gym. Ben has moved me onto 2 alternative programmes so I've got to be really clear that I know what to do – bit concerned that I didn't fully understand what I was doing yesterday.

Saturday, 28 November 2009

Two sessions with Ben again this week and as he's on holiday soon I've got to be able to follow a programme correctly on my own. Some days I stay a bit longer than the usual hour if I think I have the energy left, but should I be working harder? What I mean is, if I still have some energy left at the end of the workout then should I have put more effort into the workout itself? My programme now includes 500m of rowing as fast as I can – this is very hard!

My schedule is now – programme 1, programme 2, sprints, programme 1, programme 2, sprints, etc. It's not good to do weights every day as your body needs time to recover but I also don't think that 30 minutes of sprints is enough exercise so I think on those days I'll also go for a walk/run during the morning.

I weighed myself this morning and I weigh 2lbs less than I did this time last week which is good! What's more important is that I'm feeling slimmer, clothes are looser and I'm feeling so much healthier. I'm now going to bed earlier to give my body a chance to repair, the best sleep is between 10.30pm and 1am. I've also increased my magnesium/ zinc dose and I really am sleeping deeper now. I've also been reading up more on healthy eating, juicing and protein. This has led me to order some probiotic tablets, not the crap they sell in the supermarket which is full of sugar, but proper stuff!

Sunday, 29 November 2009

I'm really pleased with how I've been doing these past 3 days. I'm eating small meals, regularly, taking all my tablets, going to bed at 10pm, falling asleep by 10.30pm and now because I'm taking 3 magnesium tablets I'm getting deeper sleep for longer which means my body is repairing more at night. I've been highly focused at the gym and eating good food slowly. Once again, I'm back on the psyllium husk which I also feel does me a lot of good. I couldn't help but get on the scales this morning and I'm 17 stone 3. I must resist the temptation until weigh day in the future, though.

I've now planned my exercise schedule ahead until I next see Ben. I'm only going to have one day when I don't go, the day we go to Manchester to see Placebo. I want Ben to see a noticeable difference when he's back and I want to be 16 stone 07 at Christmas. I think it is a stretch with these past two weeks but I'm going to see how close I can get.

Fizzy water can leach our bodies of calcium. Ben said if I wanted sparking water it has to be naturally sparkling. Today I read the labels at the supermarket. There are two waters I can buy, one being San Pellegrino. The label says 'this is from a naturally carbonated source' but can water be naturally carbonated? I rang the help desk number and got to speak with their nutritionist. This is probably a bit obsessive, but what I want more than anything is to be fit and healthy. I remember when I first started with Ben he asked me if I wanted to lose weight quickly or get healthy. No point in being slim but unhealthy.

'The most important conversations, briefings, meeting, and lectures you will ever have will be those you hold with yourself in the privacy of your own mind.'

Denis Waitley

WEEK 9

Wednesday, 2 December 2009
Weight: 17 stone 4lbs
23lbs total loss, no change

No food since 6.20pm last night as I had a fasting insulin test this morning. I wanted to see if I am verging on diabetic and I've also had my cholesterol levels tested. I had to go straight from the doctors to the gym so there was no time for a proper breakfast, instead I decided to have a protein shake. I had a sample pack of whey protein powder and thought it would be similar to what I normally use. Big mistake – whey protein varies and this was sweet and horrible. I should have read the ingredients. It contained 5.9g of sugar per 100g and also contains a sweetener – sucralose.

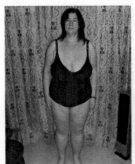
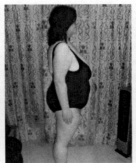
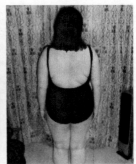

PRIORITISE

Going to the gym and cooking healthy food has to be a priority. We can spend hours watching TV and on the computer without thinking twice. We need to prioritise and decide what is important, then we will find the time. Jot down your gym schedule in your diary just as you would business appointments.

I worked hard in the gym and ate great all day. This evening I could have my carb meal. I've been missing toast and marmite so that's what I had - 2 slices plus some chips. It was good but I know I wouldn't eat this every day. I sent out my email newsletter today and told over 2000 people about my weight loss and health goals and got some great replies back. I do think telling the world is a great way of keeping me focused on my goal.

TIP: Tell people. It will help to keep you focused and holds you accountable.

Thursday, 3 December 2009

The last thing I want to do is to give the impression that I'm finding this easy. There are times when I'd like to eat, not 'bad foods', I wouldn't want to eat nasty food full of bad chemicals, but a piece of cheese, a glass of red wine and a big bowl of fruit salad – that's the sort of food I want to have, and porridge! But that's for the future. I know I could have it if I wanted, and that's why I have my carb meal on every 5th day, but if I want to get to goal as quickly as possible I've got to stay on track. Same with going to the gym, both yesterday and today I'd have been happy to stay at home and carry on working, but if I don't go Ben (my personal trainer) may ask why I didn't so it seemed easier to go!

Today after my second set of exercises I could have lied and skipped a set but I would only be cheating myself and it is a good feeling to know I did it and I made good progress today.

As you read this you may think it's easy for you Denise, paying out for a personal trainer twice a week. It comes down to priorities. I'm saving money by not buying chocolate and wine, we no longer have our regular meals out - now only very occasionally - and we've adjusted our spending so no holiday this year as we have both prioritised my health.

PERSONAL TRAINERS CAN'T DO IT FOR YOU

A trainer on its own won't make a difference. It's the commitment to healthy eating and adherence to an exercise plan that gets results.

WEEK 10

Monday, 7 December 2009
Weight: 17 stone 2lbs
25lbs total loss

With a 2lb loss since last week I should be happy but I still wanted more ... I am working out hard however so I really do think I am building muscle.

Tuesday, 8 December 2009

My schedule has been tested! Today I had a radio day in London so that's had an impact on my eating and exercise. I'm occasionally used by a company to support their marketing campaign, giving a psychological input to their work. Last night I had to catch a train to London and with a late afternoon client I only had time for a small bowl of casserole. I thought I'd be okay but when I got my complimentary drink on the train (I was on expenses and in first class) they also gave me a packet of biscuits and I ate them. I didn't want them and if I had had a decent meal I wouldn't have been tempted. I'm annoyed with myself.

I had breakfast booked at the hotel but didn't want to be tempted again so I ate the breakfast food I had brought with me - smoked mackerel and tomatoes. I was only in London for the morning and had planned to buy some lunch from M&S at Paddington for the journey home, but my train was in so I dashed for it. Lunch was almonds (I always keep nuts in my bag).

When I got home, I had more smoked mackerel with raspberries and tomatoes. We'd planned to go out for a curry tonight - Simon loves them and with me having spent the day doing media work, we wanted to have a bit of a celebration. I chose to have a poppadom with onion and yoghurt dip and then had chicken tikka with salad. I wondered about naan bread and rice and then decided why not, I've been so careful for 9 weeks that I could have a treat, I also had half a pint of lager as well. But this was a planned one off, my next carb meal won't be anything like this.

NUTS, ESPECIALLY ALMONDS

Nuts are a great source of protein and a good source of healthy fats. I mainly choose almonds. Almonds reduce the risk of heart disease, they are crammed with monounsaturated fats that help lower our LDL (bad) cholesterol levels while raising levels of HDL (good) cholesterol. They also have high levels of vitamin E, calcium and magnesium. 1 handful contains as much vitamin E as 23 handfuls of cashews! They also take longer to eat because of the outer covering and thus you use up calories just eating them. It's best to weigh out a 25g portion otherwise you may be as tempted as I am to keep dipping into the bag and eat the lot.

TIP: An occasional treat keeps motivation topped up.

Friday, 11 December 2009

Yesterday I went to the gym. I didn't want to go, I have so much work on but know I have to go and I've missed out these past two days. I'm focused on eating healthy, my 6 meals consist of 3 normal sized ones and 3 smaller helpings, I'm sure that's where I went wrong before, I stopped losing weight as I was eating too much.

HOW TO BE YOUR OWN PERSONAL TRAINER

Not everyone can afford personal trainers, not everyone wants to pay for gym visits, but we can all set ourselves goals and challenges and monitor progress. We could opt for a walking plan, buy a pedometer and note how many steps we are doing and set a plan to increase each week - both steps and the time to complete e.g. a 3 mile walk.

My tweed trousers are now getting loose on me. I also tried on my linen trousers and these fit me perfectly, they were at least 2 sizes too small when I started 10 weeks ago. Sizes are odd though. I ordered some new PJs from John Lewis in a size 20 and I thought they might be too big but they are tight on my bust so I need to put them to one side until I've lost about another 10lbs.

I got on the scales this morning and I'm 17 stone so just 1lb off the 2 stone target and I've 5lb lost in just 2 weeks, so I'm feeling very pleased.

Yesterday I did my blood test to check out if I am deficient in vitamin D, then posted the test to the US. I wonder when I'll hear about my blood tests from the doctors? It's been over a week. I've probably not heard as everything is okay but I'd like to know.

Sunday, 13 December 2009

I didn't go to the gym on Friday but I did go on Saturday and Sunday. Today it would have been so easy to stay home mooching around the house, but will that get me to my goal? No! So I went and was glad to have gone, it really gets the endorphins going.

My tidying up lead to me finding some of the meal replacement stuff I used to take - why did I? Reading the ingredients of the isotonic drink which is meant to be healthy I saw it was virtually all sugar. As I type this I'm having a healthy mini meal - some blackberries, cherry tomatoes and sesame seeds - such a change from what I'd have eaten in the past.

FOOD PLANS

We all differ and the food plan I am following may not be right for you. This book is about how one person lost nearly half of her body weight and can serve to motivate you on your own fitness journey.

The key thing to remember is that food is a fuel, and we need to eat healthily, although not to excess, and we also need to really increase our activity - not just through going to the gym but also through adding movement throughout our day.

If we are insulin resistant we need to include weight training in our exercise programme. Walking is good but it is important to build muscle, it will help to increase insulin sensitivity in the long term.

WEEK 11

Monday, 14 December 2009
Weight: 17 stone 0lbs
27lbs total loss

Another 2 pound loss, all going well. Ben took measurements again today. He reminded me to take photos - I don't like it but know I need to! We moved on to some new exercises, Ben always tests that I can do a particular exercise correctly as the worst thing is to do an exercise incorrectly. I'll now be able to include lunges.

Here you can see how my measurements have decreased, I'm very pleased with the 4cm drop on my hips.

MEASUREMENT REDUCTIONS

Bust	2cm
Biceps, right	0.5cm
Waist	1cm
Hips	4cm
Thigh, right	1cm
Calf, right	0.5cm

Thursday, 17 December 2009

I always have a protein shake straight after my workout to help with recovery. Ben joined me and we chatted about business and goal setting. So many people are putting off getting fit till after Christmas but why not get focused now? I was telling him that someone had asked me if I'd go back to 'normal eating' when I'd lost all my weight - not at all - I'm very happy to continue with my healthy life style. Ben had said that I'm quite funny, as I talk straight, but isn't that the best way? The test results have come back, and all my results are within acceptable limits. Given that I weighed over 17 stone when the tests were done this is remarkable and demonstrates the power of a healthy diet and exercise.

START TODAY

Don't wait till tomorrow, or Monday or the New Year. Today is a perfect day to start.

'Two little words that can make the difference: START NOW.'
Mary C. Crowley

Saturday, 19 December 2009

My carb day. I really fancied a cheese and pickle bread roll, so decided to have that with some tomatoes on the side. I thought it was a great idea as I hadn't had cheese or a crusty French roll for so long but actually, it wasn't that great, and I didn't finish, it was too much bread and sat heavy so I won't opt for that again. We ate healthily for tea - duck and veggies - but then mid evening I had a real desire for a glass of wine and ended up drinking more than half a bottle, wondering if it was the bread that set me off? This is the first time I've gone off plan but I have also been so busy that maybe I needed to relax and alcohol is my drug.

CHRISTMAS

Most people put on 7-10 pounds at Christmas. We need to plan and think about the impact of eating what we like for a week or two. It will probably take a month (or more) to lose the weight, is it worth it? We can cut back in advance, lose a few pounds in November, then during the party season we can exercise control most of the time, perhaps choosing just one event a week where we will relax and eat what we want. When I went out to parties I always ate at home first to stop me being tempted.

Sunday, 20 December 2009

I have been strict with food today and did a full workout at the gym today. The lunges are quite hard on my weak leg (we all have one leg that is stronger than another) but I persevered and did more than last time.

WEEK 12

Monday, 21 December
Weight: 16 stone 12lbs
29lbs total loss

Another 2 pound loss and so all is going well.

Tuesday, 22 December 2009

I'm not feeling well and if I hadn't paid to see Ben would probably have skipped today, but I went, told him I didn't think I would be able to do as much yet ended up doing more! I told him about my carb day on Saturday. I had it wrong, I was meant to eat carbs after 6pm and after I'd had my normal meal. It was hard in the gym today but I was amazed at how much I did, my straight leg dead lift has increase by over 100% in a week!

Saturday, 26 December 2009

I'm happy with my eating on Christmas Day. Just as Ben recommended I ate my usual way until our evening meal, where we had guinea fowl, sprouts and I had 2 roast potatoes. I then drank over half a bottle of champagne, but this is my weakness and I'd promised myself this as a treat. It was quite icy outside so we didn't go for our planned walk up Bredon Hill but I did dance around the kitchen.

DEALING WITH SPECIAL OCCASIONS

Christmas and other special occasions can be difficult, it's hard to get the food and alcohol right and we all realise that once we start drinking alcohol it's hard to stop. One thing I was less aware of was the real damage it does to our diets. All the energy (calories) in the alcohol has to be used up before our body uses the calories from the food we have eaten. Because of this, alcohol can have a dramatically negative impact on our diet.

I'm still taking the psyllium husk, I really don't like it, but it certainly fills me up, contains no calories and helps get rid of 'waste products' in the body. Don't want to be more descriptive than that!

Sunday, 27 December 2009

I've had a healthy Christmas but haven't done any exercise for 2 days so I was looking forward to going to the gym today. This morning I went through the Flora heart age quiz - I had to enter my weight, heart, blood pressure and cholesterol scores and also my waist measurement. With my current results (including a 127cm waist; and my weight of 16 stone 9) it shows me as 44 (my real age is 53). I then did it again with my weight changed to 13 stone and a 101.5cm (40 inch) waist and finally with a weight of 9 stone 13 and a waist of 65.5cm (27 inches) and nothing changes! Not sure how accurate this is. Seems to be more like a magazine quiz.

WEEK 13

Monday, 28 December 2009
Weight: 16 stone 7lbs
34lbs total loss

I've lost five pounds over Christmas, which is truly remarkable when most people will put this and more on. I'm now only one lb away from losing two and a half stone overall. Will I lose that by tomorrow? Probably not, but even so that amounts to 34lbs in 13 weeks which is more than 2lbs a week so overall I'm delighted.

I'm still drinking lots of water. Drinking a litre for every 50 pounds of body weight means that I need to drink just over 4.5 litres (8 pints) and this is in addition to the water I drink at the gym.

Wednesday, 30 December 2009

I had such a busy day yesterday with lots of radio interviews and no time to eat, so I had eggs for breakfast, just a protein shake for lunch, a slice of ham and some nuts after the gym and smoked mackerel and carrots for tea then blueberries later. I also had a glass of wine with my evening meal, I did this for a treat because today had been stressful.

HEALTHY EATING CAN BE QUICK

Twice a week I cook up a big pan of stew and save portions in the freezer.

I worked out with Ben yesterday and the day before that I just did sprints - I must only do 2 consecutive days of weights and I'd forgotten about that as I was so eager to do well.

'Success is often achieved by those who don't know that failure is inevitable.'

Coco Chanel, fashion designer

Saturday, 2 January 2010

I was invited to a large family lunch yesterday. This led to a dilemma. I had to decide whether to go along and eat what I was given or to make it clear what I could/couldn't eat. I had a small bowl of homemade soup followed by two small potatoes with my meal. I skipped the honey roasted veggies and also the desserts - I'd taken my own strawberries! My weakness was a glass and a half of wine but this was my carb meal so it was okay. Everyone commented on how well I looked, so how great will I look in 6 months time when we have our party? I should be another 3 stone lighter and I will be looking really good by then!

I continue to take my psyllium husk after each meal and next week I'll be back on the apple fibre.

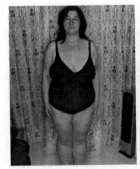 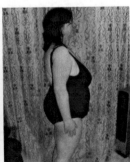 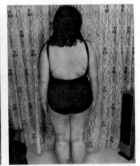

WEEK 14

Monday, 4th January 2010
Weight: 16 stone 6lbs
35lbs total loss

Looking back on New Year I think I was being a bit of a zealot not eating the honey covered veggies but I did drink wine. My results speak volumes however and I have lost two and a half stone since I started by remaining disciplined.

I have now set myself a weekly target from now until my summer party. To lose 2.5lbs a week. I've created a chart to monitor my progress - I know you shouldn't weigh yourself too often but yesterday morning I got on the scales and had put on a pound. I don't weigh my foods but almonds are calorie dense and I'm probably eating too many. Today I was much happier to be at 16 stone 5.

Ben has encouraged me to juice veggies. He suggests, nutritionally speaking, that green vegetables are best. I tried all sorts although I'm really not sure how you are meant to get juice out of cauliflower, broccoli or cabbage. Celery had far too much of a salty taste but cucumber has been fine.

JUICING VEGGIES

We should increase the amount of raw food in our diets. Juicing vegetables is a great way to do this. Cucumber has a lot of water and is easy to juice and okay to drink. The first glass or two had a weird taste but I soon became accustomed to this. I have found that taking it first thing in the morning makes me feel healthy and virtuous. We get a major jolt of vitamins and many supplements are also derived from green vegetables.

Wednesday, 6 January 2010

Heavy snow today meant I couldn't get to the gym or even go out for a walk so no exercise and too much temptation to eat. I'm also quite down because of some personal difficulties, it is horrible when someone is hurtful to you but this time I've endured the pain rather than mask it with food and drink.

I had quite a few client enquiries so I was kept busy with them and ongoing projects but there was a temptation to eat so I decided this should be my carb day. This was fair as my last one was New Years Day. I had a jacket potato and a protein flapjack and a couple of glasses of wine. When I went to bed I could really tell I'd been drinking, I had more than I should have had. However, when I felt low in the past I would have pigged out on chocolate and I didn't do that today and it's important that I am kind to myself from time to time.

ALCOHOL

Alcohol tastes nice but we need to think of the impact it has on our body. It is a toxin that puts strain on our liver, kidneys and more. It triggers insulin secretion and increases body fat storage. It is also full of empty calories. Our body needs to use up the calories from alcohol before it burns the calories from other food so even protein can turn to fat in it's presence. It really is a toxic substance and a depressant too!

Friday, 8 January 2010

I know I did very little exercise yesterday, my step counter showed about 1500 steps which is appalling, but I just wasn't feeling up to dancing. I'm glad I got to the gym today but it is odd training without

Ben. Today was great, several of the staff from the gym told me how well I'm doing. Adam (a PT) said he wished that everyone was as motivated as me! I might not have lost any weight today but having lost 6lb in the past two weeks I'm okay with this as I know I've been doing all the right things. I juiced my first cucumber today and all went really well.

DANCING IN THE KITCHEN

When you wear a pedometer, it's really easy to add a few hundred steps here and there. I like to dance around the kitchen when I'm cooking! You might think I'm odd but it's all about getting moving.

WEEK 15

Monday, 11 January 2010
Weight: 16 stone 6lbs
35lbs total loss, no change

I'm now getting fed up of the snow and bad weather. The worst part is that I'm having clients postpone and they are backing up! On Saturday I went to the gym and did sprints, hadn't done them for 3 weeks and it was tough so I should probably do these each week. This time I stepped up my running pace to 9.5kph. We had friends around on Saturday evening so I planned what to eat and drink.

PREPARE IN ADVANCE

Plan in advance for those days when your motivation is going to be tested. I thought about how best to handle having friends around and decided to drink sparkling mineral water and eat the crusty bread and cheese as my treat.

By late Sunday morning I was feeling a bit grumpy and on edge and not sure why. It might have been because I had a never ending pile of work on my desk. Simon cooked a perfect breakfast - scrambled eggs with tomatoes and mushrooms - but as we were going to the cinema I ended up having a rushed lunch, basically just grabbing half a portion of chicken and some celery. After the cinema I was so hungry that I bought a bag of cashew nuts. Got home and thought I'd be okay till our evening meal but felt empty, I don't know what it was about yesterday but cheese called for me - 4 different cheeses in the fridge was too much of a temptation so I decided I would have some bread and cheese, then I had 2 glasses of white wine as well.

After 14 weeks of staying focused I think it's fine to go off plan for an occasional meal but this wasn't planned, this was being driven by cravings.

This morning the scales flickered between 16 stone 06 and 16 stone 07 but settled on 16 stone 06 so no change. After going to the gym today and eating 'clean' I should lose this pound but my hopes of getting to 16 stone by Friday have been dashed, I think this is going to be impossible.

In yesterday's Sunday Times I read about the 10 best fitness websites. What interested me was the link to Men's Health, lots of interesting articles and not just for men. I also went to www.djsteveboy.com/podrunner.html where you can download dance mixes that are high energy to help get you through a workout.

WEEK 16

Monday, 18 January 2010
Weight: 16 stone 6lbs
35lb loss, no change

I haven't lost weight in the past 2 weeks. I feel better about it than the last time I plateaued but I wonder why? I know that people aren't machines and that we can't expect consistent progress. I also know that the scales are only one measurement and progress is also to do with what you look like, how you feel and what your other measurements are.

I've also looked inwards and know there are things I did which may have contributed to my plateau - I ate bread and cheese on Saturday, far too many nuts, skipped going to the gym. Plus, Simon found some of the 'Eat Natural' small yoghurt covered bars in the cupboard and I think I ate three. As they were still in the cupboard I ate a couple more this week. There was also the wine on Sunday night - only 2 small glasses, but even so...

I'm wondering ... I kept so focused for 14 weeks and in the past few days I think I reached the point that lots of us reach where we just want to eat the things we want. I know I have my carb meal every 5 days and think I could have been better with my food, so I consider this setback a lesson learned.

On the plus side, the personal trainers at the gym are saying that I'm like a different person and that I look great.

LACK OF FOCUS

Sometimes it is easy to slip and to wonder why we have plateaued. When I faced up to myself I realised it was because there was a loss of focus. There has been stress in my private life and stress can lead to us holding onto weight but I also ate more - flapjacks, bread and cheese etc.

Thursday, 21 January 2010

Today was my monthly measurement day. Look at the chart below to see how much I have lost.

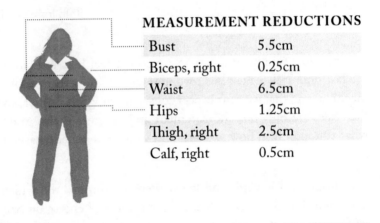

MEASUREMENT REDUCTIONS

Bust	5.5cm
Biceps, right	0.25cm
Waist	6.5cm
Hips	1.25cm
Thigh, right	2.5cm
Calf, right	0.5cm

So I'm still moving forwards and I'm pleased I did such a great work out today. I've progressed from 4 sets of 12 squats with 6kg in each hand to 4 sets of 20 with 8kg in each hand. I am now dead lifting 37.5kg instead of 32.5kg. So onwards, I'll continue with what I'm doing and aim for a 3lb loss next week!

Friday, 22 January 2010

Since Friday I have been strict and I have been eating clean, cutting back on the amount of nuts I've been eating. However, I've only been to the gym once this week. After working hard for days on end I took Saturday off - I was busy, had a client with me for over 3 hours. I then went shopping and to the cinema. The next day I was fine when I woke up but after sitting at my desk for 3 hours I stood up and my back hurt. I didn't think that much of it and I still went to the gym but in the evening my back really started to hurt and on Monday was even worse - so I have used ice, heat and massage and although I am in a lot less pain it's still tender so I won't go back to the gym till Tuesday. It's been very weird, not working out, but the last thing I want to do is to damage my back.

Sunday, 23 January 2010

We went to Blackpool to see The Prodigy on Saturday. Figuring out what I'm going to eat when we are away is hard so this time we bought food from M&S and had a picnic in our hotel room. As we had some free time we did some shopping and I tried on clothes. I bought two size 18 tops and both fitted well. I also tried on some size 18 cargo trousers, these had no stretch and were tight in the leg and were a slightly stretched hand width too small across my belly. I thought this was a useful yardstick and I'll go in to the store once I've lost another stone to see how they then fit. On Sunday we met family, and went out for a Chinese meal. It was a buffet and it was hard to know what to eat. I had some of the sweet and sour pork and a small helping of rice and noodles but this was my carb day so it was allowed.

WEEK 17

Monday, 25 January 2010
Weight: 16 stone 2lbs
39lbs total loss

Wow, I was 16 stone and 06lbs this time last week and this week I'm 16 stone 02lbs. I'm amazed. It was with much hesitation that I got on the scales this morning and I was flabbergasted to find that I'd lost 4lb, so feeling very happy!

I wrote last week that there are many different measures of progress and weight is just one of them, but it is still great to see a loss on the scales, especially as without exercise I've not had the benefit of using up more calories. It just goes to show that there isn't a strict, linear relationship between food/exercise and weight. Things aren't that simple.

Wednesday, 27 January 2010

A day in London where I still managed to 'eat clean' and my second day back at the gym - 10 days spent without a workout had me wondering what it would be like to return to the gym. Everything was fine, although yesterday I was very wobbly doing my first set of split lunges. Today I did deadlifts but only did 10 or 13 reps, decided not to push myself too much.

Friday, 29 January 2010

Yesterday and today I worked out with Ben. He pushed me so hard yesterday and my legs hurt so much - overall I did 80 split lunges (4 x 20) and on everything else I was pushed to my limit, but it is paying off!

Sunday, 31 January 2010

Yesterday I had my carb evening meal and I consciously chose what to eat and drink. I had half a bottle of champagne, some pineapple, 2 mini yoghurt covered bars and a piece of french bread. This was more than I normally have but I decided I would treat myself, it was just for one meal, and the 2 mini bars were in the cupboard ... otherwise I wouldn't have had them. I went to the gym this afternoon and worked hard. I didn't go to the gym yesterday in order to give my body a chance to recover and build.

WHAT'S IN THE STORE CUPBOARD?

We get tempted when we have food in our cupboards. Having biscuits, crisps, bottles of wine or cider at home can lead us to succumb to temptation. It is far better to remove any of these items. My husband loves pork pie, and I like it too, so I was a bit bossy and made him eat it away from home. If you think you can't resist, don't buy it in the first place.

'The question isn't who is going to let me; it's who is going to stop me.'

Ayn Rand

WEEK 18

Monday, 1 February 2010
Weight: 15 stone 11lbs
44lbs total loss

Woo hoo! I'm 15 stone 11 today. Last week I was 16 stone and 2 pounds so this means I've lost 5lbs this week and 9lbs overall in the past fortnight, however prior to this I had a 2 week plateau so this means I have lost 9lbs in the past month which is a good result anyway. But this week? Who knows why I've dropped so much: I spent 9 days without going to the gym or doing much exercise due to my bad back but this week I have had plenty of juiced vegetables and I've eaten good, clean food. For example, yesterday I juiced half a cucumber and later half a head of celery. I've also started measuring out nuts, so I know roughly how many I can eat

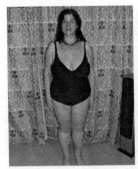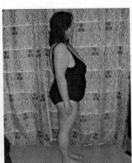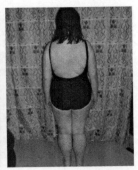

for about 150 calories which is much better than having a 100 gram bag which I dip into.

The great thing about losing weight is that my husband notices! After 13 years of marriage, things go a bit – well, you know - but now he loves putting his hands around me and they now overlap rather than stretch to meet and he comments about how much better I look. Bless him.

As usual he made me a lovely breakfast - scrambled eggs and grilled mushrooms. I had a few nuts mid morning and I've just juiced half a cucumber, this gives me such an energy boost and I don't know why other people don't juice.

I'm not looking forward to going away tonight. I've got 2 days of consultancy work ahead and not only do I hate being away from home but there is also the concern about food. I'm having to take my own food rather than rely on the food that is provided. I'm not even sure if I can have the breakfast. I know they have fruit salad but I can only eat berries. I'll ask them to give me a bowl of strawberries and 2 boiled eggs, but will they?

Wednesday, 3 February 2010

The second day of working in London I decided to skip breakfast and get to the office really early. I then had some chicken, carrot sticks and tomatoes plus nuts so that was lunch and breakfast sorted. Yesterday many people commented on how good I was looking; I also demonstrated the depth of squats I can do! There's a big pile of biscuits near the drinks machine and I wasn't tempted at all, whereas previously I'd have eaten lots - they are in packets of 3, and being honest I could easily have gone through 3 packets in a day if not 4. Same in the hotel, there were 2 packets of biscuits plus a big plate of fruit, but nothing was on my list of food to eat. I was also able to be strict for breakfast - picking strawberries out of the fruit salad and asking for 2 hard boiled eggs.

Once back with Simon we went out for a meal. I took my carb meal a day early but I hardly went mad: I ate one poppadom with onion and yoghurt dip then had chicken tikka with some spinach and cheese, a quarter plate of rice and about a quarter of a naan bread plus a quarter pint of beer.

Thursday, 4 February 2010

I had a facial and a massage first thing which meant I was tired for most of the day. Not the best time of day to have one. Jo, my beauty therapist, couldn't believe how much I've shrunk and she noticed that my skin is tightening up, too. It was meant to be a quiet day but I have taken on 3 new clients so plenty of talking and organising. I saw Ben at 4pm and I had a new workout, gosh I had to struggle through some of this! At the gym Ben asked me to pick up a 20kg weight, it was so very hard. He then said 'that's how much you've lost'. It really brought home to me how much extra I was carrying around with me.

Friday, 5 February 2010

This morning I put my jeans on. These have lycra in them and are usually a real stretch to get on after being washed. Today I didn't even have to hold in to get the zip up so these will be in the fat ladies pile shortly. When I get close to 15 stone, maybe in 3 weeks, I'm going to go back to M&S to retry on the cargo pants. I think this is a great way to spot any differences without buying new clothes. I weighed 14 stone when I met Simon and I was in size 18 clothes then. This was when I didn't do any exercise so I'm sure I'll find the 18s are comfortable at 15 stone and by the time our party comes around I might even find size 16s are loose. I can't imagine wearing size 14s again - that will be brilliant.

I'm about to buy tickets for us to go to Rockness. I must have weighed around 18 stone when we went last year, maybe more, as it was June and the weight was going up. I'm going to look so much better and I wonder if I will fit into normal wellies? I had to buy snow boots which I only wear because they are wide enough for my calves.

I do like having my cucumber before breakfast; it really makes me feel healthy. Ben has suggested juicing cauliflower, I'm not sure, I can't actually imagine it. Maybe I need to buy a book on juicing combinations. I probably need to create my own.

WEEK 19

Monday, 8 February 2010
Weight: 15 stone 09lbs
46lbs total loss

Result! Another 2lb loss, bringing me down to 15 stone 09. I was a bit concerned I'd have remained static as I did eat 70gms of nuts yesterday but everything else I ate was quite light and that's probably why I needed the nuts.

Thursday, 11 February 2010

I've been so busy with the launch of my third book, *'Now you've been shortlisted'*, as well as with my usual client work that I haven't had a moment to write this diary. I also had to skip going to the gym yesterday as there is too much to do. I've eaten more nuts than I should but I haven't gone off the plan. I've also not been going to bed as early as I should have been and I think my period is due, all of which doesn't bode well for losing weight this week.

This afternoon I had a session with Ben. It was hard going, but I did it! We finished 5 minutes early so Ben suggested I have my protein drink and watch him demonstrate how to do an exercise, no bench to sit on so I squatted, Ben said that I can squat better than him, I'm used to squatting from when I used local toilets whilst travelling in India!

FOLLOW WHAT WORKS

Ben said that the reason I've been so successful is that I do exactly what I'm told both in the gym and at home. I have a plan and (for the majority of the time) I follow it. I hope my story has been inspiring you so far.

Friday, 12 February 2010

Measurement day at the gym and Ben was amazed at the drop in measurements; the changes are as good as last month.

MEASUREMENT REDUCTIONS

Bust	4.5cm
Biceps, right	0.25cm
Waist	2.5cm
Hips	8.25cm
Thigh, right	2.75cm
Calf, right	0.5cm

Ben was featured in the local paper a couple of weeks ago and they included a photo of me, one of his star clients. This lead to Ben taking on a new client who read about my story. Today my weight was only down by half a pound but I'm not distraught this time as I know weight is but one measurement of progress. Also, I have been quite stressed and I haven't been getting to bed as early as I would like. Both may affect weight loss. I've been so busy today that I didn't have time for lunch, what with clients virtually back to back, so I ended up snacking on nuts all day. Not ideal.

STRESS CAN MAKE US FAT

There are many types of stress. Stress can be caused by emotional, hormonal or physical triggers such as being too hot or cold (thermic). When we are stressed our body releases cortisol and this can lead to fat accumulation around our middle and makes it very difficult to reduce levels of fat as our body switches to a 'slow setting'. I used alcohol and carbs as my drug of choice for dealing with stress but as you've seen exercising and relaxing is a much better way of fighting back.

Saturday, 13 February 2010

I've had two clients here today so it's been busy but I had half of a large cucumber early in the morning and the other half when I got back from the gym so I've had lots of nutrients today. I worked hard at the gym and we concentrated on arm exercises with weights, a brilliant way to get rid of bingo wings.

Sunday, 14 February 2010

Today I looked through my online photos and found some photos of me at my biggest, I'd forgotten how enormous I was. Back then I really was one of those greatly overweight people that others stare at whereas at the moment I look like someone within a normal range - still heavy, but because I'm toned, I look okay. I don't just want to look okay, however, I want to look fantastic!

I've been working it out and I have realised that I first started my weight loss campaign back in April 2004, that's when the person who sold me meal replacement powders got in contact and back then I knew I had to do something. So although these chapters may make my weight loss seem easy, there have been many set backs along the way. With that said, I have been very focused for the past 5 months.

Today was the day of my carb meal, so a bottle of champagne shared with Simon plus a few chips with my tea and 2 crackers with stilton.

WEEK 20

Monday, 15 February 2010
Weight: 15 stone 7lbs
48lbs total loss

Whoop! whoop! Got on the scales this morning and I've lost 2lbs in the past week, (so now only 2lbs to go) until I've lost 50lbs since October and made a 100lb loss since my fattest. I want to be there by next Friday - it will be such a brilliant achievement.

Here's me thinking I look good, but having reviewed my latest photos, I still look fat. Is this motivating or depressing, I'm not sure? I saw an ad for a well known fast food chain and it reminded me that so many adverts and packaging say something like: 'Good for you as part of a calorie controlled diet', but this isn't true, it's not good food and it leads to further temptation.

WE NEED GOOD NUTRITION

It's important to eat highly nutritious food. When we focus on points and calorie counting we can eat poor quality food.

Thursday, 19 February 2010

Yesterday Emma gave me a big hug and called me slim. Clearly I'm not, but we both know how much better I look. She also said that Ben is very proud of me.

Today I did my work out with Ben and it was hard. I followed programme 12 for the last time and Ben upped the weights some more. I'm now using the metal bar to lift weights as it is easier than holding a dumbbell in each hand. I've also been doing squats with a 6kg kettle bell. Usually, I had to walk over to the bike after this which gave me a bit of a break. Not today, we took the kettle bell right over to the bike so I barely got a break. I thought I would collapse and I had to do three iterations of this cycle. My legs were like jelly at the end. Ben said this is the sort of exercise you give to personal trainers you don't like as it was such a hard one, I really don't think I could have done any more!

COMMITMENT

> Is the hardest part getting to the gym? No, it's being fully committed to working out to the max. Showing up and going through the motions is not enough. No one can do it for me, I have to give 100% to each exercise.

Saturday, 20 February 2010

What a hard day at the gym yesterday, I really can't believe what Ben put me through and it made me feel sick at one point, apparently that's a good sign though. Ben had me doing split squats with 5kg in each hand, then some bent over rows with 8kg weights, which seemed easy by comparison, then the killer, squatting with a 6kg kettle bell and then lifting the bell into the air - phew, I felt like collapsing. This was followed with time on the rowing machine.

Ben said this was advanced stuff, and that it's great for burning fat. Maybe he has put me onto this as I haven't lost any weight this week. I have lost 11lb over the past 3 weeks, though, so I'm not distraught about this.

Last night we went for dinner at Carol and Hugh's. We had a lovely time and because this was my carb meal I was able to eat what I was given, vegetable soup and bread, but the main course - chicken stuffed with camembert and covered with bacon - was very rich. I had plenty of veggies but I was careful with the potato and celeriac mash as I saw how much butter and cream went into this.

I also had 2 glasses of sparkling wine, which I drank quickly. I do find it hard to just have one glass of wine, not sure how to pace myself, better to just say no perhaps?

Today I've been so very tired, I need to have a decent night's sleep. Because I'm tired I've felt hungry so I've snacked on nuts and eaten about 400cals worth, so a good food but too much of it.

WHEN WE ARE TIRED

When we are tired we often crave high fat foods. These increase our blood sugar levels and give us a sugar high which is then followed by a sugar low, making us feel even more tired. It is far better to eat clean food at regular intervals.

Simon has been in the loft and got out my old bag of size 18 clothes. I'm not there yet, I need to lose at least another 2" all over, bit depressing really, but these clothes don't have any stretch to them. Also, I remember that these are the clothes I wore when I weighed 14 stone, which is about 20lbs less than where I am now. They are now hanging in my wardrobe so I have them ready. I've also gone through and put in the 'get rid of pile' all those round neck t shirts that clearly aren't a good look for me.

TIP: Don't skip meals - that's why I eat every 3 hours.

Sunday, 21 February 2010

My legs still ache, I worked so hard on Friday and I don't feel any better today, possibly even worse, so I'm not sure how I'm going to be at the gym today as I've never felt so sore after an exercise session before. My legs and bottom hurt so much that it is hard to get up the stairs or even to get on the loo!

WEEK 21

Monday, 22 February 2010
Weight: 15 stone 4lbs
51lbs total loss

A 3 pound loss. The past 5 weeks have been great, I've lost 1st 2lb and I've now lost 101lbs overall! Woo! Looking back in my diary, I've lost 16lbs since I bought a dress at M&S and tried on some size 18 cargo pants which were too small. I must try them on again next week. Last week was tough with my new programme. It's a tough workout but that means it is doing me good.

CHANGING EXERCISES

Our body adapts quickly to exercise and then it's not doing us much good. That's why my personal trainer changes what I do on a regular basis. Gyms employ fitness instructors who will create a programme for you and show you what to do, but it will be down to you to ask for it to be updated regularly.

I've been so busy with work it has been hard to update this diary. On Tuesday I had to travel to London to record a podcast for The Guardian. I took 2 hard boiled eggs for my breakfast and just drank water. This time I noticed all the large people struggling to get down the aisle in the standard class carriage, I used to be like that, bumping into the people sat down, but not any more. Now I don't have a problem going down the aisles and I was even able to get out of my seat with the drop down table down. There was a very large lady sat across the aisle from me who went to buy a muffin and a sandwich. When I was fat I would never eat in public, I never wanted people making comments on the fat person eating fattening food. I noticed her and within about 30 minutes she was eating chocolate and then sweets. Clearly she wasn't hungry but her body was seeking nourishment and told her to eat more and more till it got it.

It was the same at the cinema last night. I saw a very large couple; she bought large popcorn and coke, he was buying the pick n mix. They'll still be hungry when they leave after such unhealthy food.

BREAKING THE HABIT

Often we eat and drink out of habit. An example of this is eating chocolates or popcorn and having a fizzy drink at the cinema. We need to break these habits, perhaps taking chewing gum instead of sweets or sharing a small popcorn rather than having a large bucket to ourselves.

Saturday, 27 February 2010

We went to London for the weekend as I had a work assignment on Monday, we decided to buy me some new clothes. First of all we looked in the Monsoon store at Paddington Station. I wanted to show Simon a dress I liked and I'd love to wear at the party, but what size to get? I can't buy it yet. I saw a lovely red coat and thought about it. We checked into the hotel and then got a bus to Marble Arch and started walking down Oxford Street. The first shop we went into was Wallis and it was nice to look at clothes and choose what I wanted to try on rather than be stuck with what I think will fit me. I bought 2 dresses, both are very flattering. We then went onto Monsoon and I bought a coat. Later Simon bought some clothes in Gap so I got changed and dumped my old baggy coat. I look so much better in my new clothes. That evening I had my scheduled carb meal in an Indian restaurant including naan bread, rice and beer.

Sunday, 28 February 2010

It was cold and wet when we woke up. We went to the National Portrait Gallery and then did more shopping. In M&S I tried on the famous size 18 cargo trousers once again. When I tried these on in Blackpool there was a several inch gap across my belly, this time they did up, just. I also tried a M&S size 18 coat on, this was too small, so although I'm a size 18 in some clothes, certainly not in all. This means I'm a size 18/20 at the moment, what I want is to be a size 12/14.

We had tickets for the theatre - Cuban music and dancing at Sadlers Wells. It was very cold in the theatre so when we got to the restaurant I was very hungry and got stuck into the bread. As we were on holiday I thought I'd go for a 2nd carb meal. We had a bottle of Prosecco, shared whitebait to start with, then had some tuna and green beans and finished with sticky toffee pudding and ice cream. A treat as it's holiday time, but on reflection I could have made better choices here.

AT RESTAURANTS

Restaurants will automatically bring us bread and we can start eating it without thinking. As soon as they bring the bread it's best to send it away to save our selves from being tempted.

'Believe you can and you're halfway there.'

Theodore Roosevelt

WEEK 22

Monday, 1 March 2010
Weight: 15 stone 4lbs
51lbs total loss, no change

A day of consultancy and meeting people I hadn't seen for a while. People commented on how great I looked, which I did! We are provided with lunch from Prêt but as I can't eat sandwiches and know the salads they provide don't contain enough protein I took along my own food - nipped into M&S and bought some thin turkey slices and cherry tomatoes. Only later did I realise that the meat contained preservatives. Ideally, I should have brought cooked chicken from home but it wouldn't have been practical as I stayed overnight in a

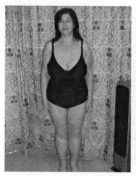 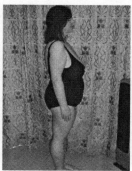 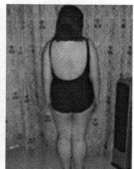

hotel. During times like these I need to compromise and this was a reasonably good choice.

Friday, 5 March 2010

Today at the hairdressers, Charlotte, my colourist, was amazed at how different I looked and I do like the way I look in my new dress and coat. I'm wearing the turquoise mac and brightly coloured dress I bought in London. I always used to wear dark clothes, thinking this would make me look smaller, but they just made me look miserable. I suit colour.

I got on the scales this morning and I'm at 15 stone 04 so no change since this time last week – I can probably attribute this to the 2 days of eating carbs. Okay, lesson learned. I know you shouldn't weigh yourself every day as there will always be fluctuations but I so hoped to have lost a pound. I'm going to have to stay focused for all my life or else I'll be putting the weight back on.

Today I wanted to eat carbs and I knew I couldn't. It really isn't easy staying focused, but as I've said before I'm in this for the long term and I've got to focus on what I need rather than what I want. I now realise that there is no way I can go back to old eating habits, I'm really going to have to stay focused on eating healthily, otherwise the weight will pile back on and that is such a waste of energy.

Saturday, 6 March 2010

We went to see my niece today and she was amazed at how I looked and really noticed when she put her arms around me as I have lost so much. In my new clothes I really look good and I will look even better with another 3 stone off me. I'm only 3lbs off losing a total of 4 stone since October. Will I be able to crack this in time for next weekend?

Simon puts his arm around my waist much more than he used to, and I let him. Previously I would have pulled away as I was so conscious of the fat around my middle.

WEEK 23

Monday, 8 March 2010
Weight: 15 stone 2lbs
53lbs total loss

Pleased to have dropped 2lbs in a week. I thought that my weight might stick as I've got a lot of stressful things going on in my personal life and I know that stress can lead to the production of cortisol and that can lead to fat gain. I may be stressed but I'm not binging on food.

BREATHING

It helps to breathe deeply. Previously when I was stressed I would calm myself down by eating high fat food such as chocolate. As I made changes I remembered the stress management technique I used to teach others about breathing properly. What I do is - breathe in for 4 seconds, hold for 8 seconds and then breathe out for 16 seconds. Doing this 5 times can really help us to deal with stressful situations and it's much better than turning to chocolate, pizza or crisps!

Friday, 12 March 2010

It's been a busy week, I've had my mum staying with us. My personal stress has continued, I'm not going into detail here, but I am concerned that the stress is interfering with my weight loss. It doesn't help as I keep crying.

I saw Ben today and had my measurements taken.

MEASUREMENT REDUCTIONS

Bust	1.75cm
Biceps, right	0cm
Waist	1.5cm
Hips	0cm
Thigh, right	1.25cm
Calf, right	0.5cm

This progress isn't bad but it's not as great as the progress I've made in the past couple of months. Progress should be expected to slow down, however, as the less weight we have to lose the harder it gets. I'm working so hard and these drops are no where near what I have been getting. I can easily get disappointed and low and this is how I feel at the moment, focusing more on where I wish I was rather than to be happy about where I am.

I liked the big drops in weight and measurements as they were motivational. I know it is unrealistic to expect that pace to continue indefinitely, though. I know I should focus more on other improvements like feeling much more healthy and being able to sit more comfortably on a bus seat. I'd forgotten about that, how awful it was on a tube or bus, knowing that I was taking up more than my share of a seat. On a bus I preferred to sit in the aisle seat so I could spill over into the aisle and on the tube I would stay standing, even if I was tired and really wanted to sit down. Rather do that than be glared out for taking more than my share of the seat.

I know I will become a fit and healthy version of me eventually and if the journey takes longer it will still be fine. I'm just impatient for success!

I kept focused on my food and exercise all week but today was carb day and I decided to have a good evening. We went out for a meal with my mum and Roger and Simon agreed to drive home so I could have a drink. Thinking back, I drank too much, we had 2 bottles of wine between 3 of us. I'm better when it is just the 2 of us where I have half a bottle of wine. I also ate bread on arrival, had pate, chips with my main course and crème brule for pudding. So much more than I usually have for a carb meal. It's occasions like this which are the most challenging and I failed to plan.

> ## CARBOHYDRATES AREN'T BAD, BUT WE NEED TO BE CAREFUL
>
> It's all but too easy to eat too many carbs, We need to eat enough to fuel our body but not so much that we lay down fat. Athletes need lots of carbs ... most people need to eat much less. Farmers feed cattle lots of carbs to fatten them up.

WEEK 24

Monday, 15 March 2010
Weight: 15 stone 03lbs
52lbs total loss, 1lb gain

On the scales this morning and my weight has jumped up by a pound. I think this is common after a carb day. I will check again in a couple of days time. I completed 3 consecutive days at the gym so I took a rest day yesterday as rest is important when it comes to lifting weights. I still wanted some exercise though so when we went to the cinema we parked the car about half a mile away so I managed to include a brisk walk in my day.

I've got a busy day today and although I planned for this, I'm still not going to be able to get to the gym today, I really just can't fit it in. Instead, I will manage a walk to 'the bend' and back, that's about a mile each way.

I do still have a lot of stress due to personal stuff and I wonder whether this is affecting my stress levels and hence my weight. I know I should stay calm but the stressful thoughts keep coming into my head. I've been incredibly careful with food today and went to bed hungry so I'm hoping for a drop when I get on the scales tomorrow.

As I lose weight I have been able to drink a bit less water. Drinking a litre for every 50 pounds of body weight means that at 15 stone I need to drink 4.2 litres, (over 7 pints) and this is in addition to the water I drink at the gym.

STAYING CALM

When we are stressed there are different approaches to staying calm. When I'm being rational I know what to do - think about why I'm feeling stressed, think about the different approaches I can take and choose which will be the most appropriate. So, I could decide to scream out loud (my mum does this!), to kick a box, to do some exercise, to focus on my breathing (this is my first choice), practice EFT (tapping based on emotional freedom technique) or eat and drink fattening food. On occasion it can be fine to think 'sod it' and knock back the wine and chocolate, but this is not the best choice. I'd rather use the wine and chocolate as a treat I consume consciously rather than as something I stuff my face with when I'm out of control.

Tuesday, 16 March 2010

On the scales this morning and I've put on another pound, so today I'm 15 stone 4 pounds. I keep thinking that stress must be to blame for this. I hope this is causing me to hold onto fluid rather than to physically put weight on. I know there is a connection with stress levels and weight gain. I'm also not getting enough sleep, with personal problems making me incredibly sad and preventing me from sleeping well. It's rare for me to wake up in the night but this has been happening recently.

STRESS LEADS TO WEIGHT GAIN

Ben confirmed that it is very common for stress to hinder weight loss. It causes fat accumulation around the stomach. Poor sleep patterns also negatively affect blood sugar regulation, making us twice as likely to gain fat.

Wednesday, 17 March 2010

I spoke to Emma at the end of my gym session and told her about the weight gain. She said that I won't have put on fat but my body will be holding fluid and if I stop thinking and worrying it will soon dissipate!

Friday, 19 March 2010

I'm back on the psyllium husk which is good at clearing out my bowels. I've also been very strict with regards to food and I've been working hard at the gym. Yesterday I was doing more advanced split squats and doing wide grip squat bar lifts which Ben says he doesn't give to anyone else.

Ben has told me that I need to take my carbs after my normal meal, I remember him saying this, so you eat chips or a jacket potato after a typical meal. I haven't been doing this, instead, I've been combining it with my meal. As I've now got exactly 3 months till our summer party I want to do everything possible to get as close as possible to a further 2 stone weight loss, or to drop 2 dress sizes. That's what I really want, to be wearing size 14 clothes, I can't remember when I could last fit into clothes of that size.

Sunday, 21 March 2010

I took a day off yesterday to allow my body to rest and today I underwent a typical and extensive workout at the gym. It's very hard doing the elevated split squats and I needed to have something next to me to hang on to. Last night for my carb meal I again had a half bottle of champagne and later had 3 crackers with cheese. Thought afterwards that I shouldn't have had these, I'm also going to give alcohol a rest for the next few weeks as I did feel like I'd had a drink this morning. Could I keep to just one glass of wine and maybe have pineapple next time instead of cheese and crackers? You might wonder about the champagne, well if I can only drink once a week I'm going to drink what I actually want, we did get a load in at half price and it's my drink of choice!

WEEK 25

Monday, 23 March 2010
Weight: 15 stone 1lb
54lbs total loss

On the scales this morning and I've lost 2 pounds from last week. It's been a bit of a hard week with the scales going up but now that the reading is lower again I'm relieved. I don't think it does me any good to weigh myself so many times, if I'd only weighed myself today I wouldn't have gone through that worry of a weight gain. I think the weight gain was because I ate too much on my carb day.

I wasn't able to do as many deadlifts with the bar as my hands hurt, I've got calluses, so today I bought some gloves. It was tough at the gym but I think I have improved a little on the elevated split squats.

Wednesday, 24 March 2010

Today was a very busy day with work, plus we have the builders in so I didn't go to the gym. No time for walks either but I am pleased that on both Sunday and Monday I was in bed around 10pm and I am planning a similar bed time tomorrow.

I went to bed just after 10 pm last night which was good but I woke before 5am, not so good. I've had some worries over some building work, we're having a gazebo built and I misunderstood the measurements so I wanted to know if it could be made bigger. Thank goodness it can but it has been very stressful.

Sunday, 28 March 2010

Sometimes it's hard to find the time to write my diary and sometimes not much has changed. I was at the gym on Friday and Saturday and again today although today I did cardio instead of weights. I hadn't done this since mid January, I decided that I must have improved so I kept to the same speed on the treadmill but went up from 45 seconds to a minute. It was tough. I still did 200m on the rower and increased the time I spent on the bike up to a minute as well and at level 10.

Yesterday was my carb meal. I'd had smoked mackerel for breakfast but maybe that wasn't enough because by lunch time I was ravenous. We'd bought some crusty bread for Simon and I couldn't resist so had bread and cheese for lunch, I also had some bread in the evening. I should have waited till this evening, even after 6 months I can still forget what to do.

WEEK 26

Monday, 29 March 2010
Weight: 15 stone
55lbs total loss

I've lost 1 pound, that's good but not great. Mind you I have got my period so that may mean that I'm holding on to some water. But 55 pounds is 25 kg, a huge amount of weight, it's a sack of potatoes.

Wednesday, 31 March 2010

Ben is ill so I have started having personal training sessions with Emma. She has a very different approach, less heavy weights and more of an emphasis on working at a fast pace and very different exercises. It was tough, but in a good way, and she is a great motivator.

I went to Next and tried on 3 pairs of jeans and 2 jackets. All of them were size 18 and fitted me with ease. I didn't find them tight at all. What I find a little weird is that some size 18 trousers I had in the loft that I haven't worn for over 13 years are about a size small around my waist - have clothing companies changed their sizing? I decided in the end to buy some from Sainsbury's, I don't want to spend £40 on a pair of jeans that will probably only last for a couple of months. I later compared the measurements on my size 18 jeans from M&S from years ago to the sizes used now and it's true, sizes have changed and a size 16 now is a size 18 from 1996. Clothes manufacturers are into vanity sizing. I definitely need to get to a size 12, as that is what a

14 used to be, and I probably should be aiming for a size 10! Even the jeans I bought yesterday are loose today, I forgot about the stretch so I'm having to wear a belt.

Today was my carb day and I also had to collect Simon from work so we decided to go to the Thai Emerald for a meal. I had chicken satay, I love this, and we shared a chicken curry in a coconut sauce and the vegetable mix had tofu in it. We also shared a portion of rice.

TOFU

Tofu is made from soya. There are conflicting views on whether this is good or bad but I have read enough studies that it can impair weight loss that I don't want to eat it on a regular basis. Unprocessed soy is absolutely fine.

'All the adversity I've had in my life, all my troubles have strengthened me...You may not realize it when it happens, but a kick in the teeth may be the best thing in the world for you.'
Walt Disney

Friday, 2 April 2010

I had a second session with Emma yesterday and I ache so much today. I'm sure it is doing me a lot of good. However, the advice she gives me differs from Ben's which is a bit confusing. Ben had said to do weights to build muscle which burns fat but Emma says doing cardio helps with fat loss. Both are probably right. I'm feeling tired today but I did sleep well last night and as it's a non client day I can focus on dealing with various tasks that have piled up on my desk.

Saturday, 3 April 2010

An early visit to the gym. I followed Emma's programme and think I did well, I was truly exhausted by the time I finished. We have a

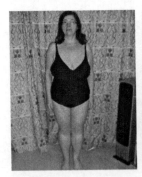 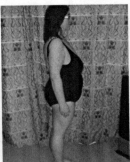 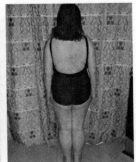

big family day tomorrow so I made one of my famous trifles. I used Madeira cake instead of Swiss roll, less chemicals in it, but there was a piece left over and I ate some. I shouldn't have, and I think I ate it on impulse. Just a small thin slice but why did I? I'd been focused earlier and said no to hot cross buns so what changed?

WEEK 27

Monday, 5 April 2010
Weight: 14 stone 13lbs
56lbs total loss

On the scales this morning and I've lost 1lb and cracked the 15 stone barrier. I thought I would have lost more but it is probably getting more difficult. It was my period last week which made me think there would be more of a drop this week. Despite having a period I think I'm going through the menopause, as my periods are sporadic and light. Luckily I don't have any bad symptoms which I think I can put down to my healthy eating.

Eight for lunch yesterday plus baby Jack so no time to go to the gym. It's also now been 6 months since I started eating healthy! I managed to keep focused on Christmas day - the last time I dined with these kind of numbers - and today decided I would eat more. I had cauli cheese, roast potatoes, gravy and trifle, more than what I would normally eat. I also had a couple of weak gin and tonics, a glass of wine plus 2 diet caffeine free cokes. Not masses more than usual, but I also plan to have a sandwich for my tea. This was all done consciously and I'll be more focused for the next 6 days.

Umm in the evening I had a glass of wine and a couple of small slices of ginger cake - I'll be back on track tomorrow.

I think this is an example of me giving in to a craving. Usually I stay strong but the longer I am focused the harder it gets. I'm usually good at not succumbing to temptation but every now and again I do, often on my carb days!

There was some left over cauli cheese so I had that with my evening meal,but apart from that I stuck with my plan.

Friday, 9 April 2010

27 weeks! I have been following my plan for a long time, but then again, the weight took a long time to add up in the first place.

Emma, my new personal trainer, has a different approach to Ben but I don't think that's a bad thing, good to give my body a bit of a shake up. Now I'm doing more cardio and sweating a heck of a lot more. Still using weights but also moving fast. Some of it is pretty hard going, swinging an 8kg medicine ball with lifts and squats. I'm also doing brand new exercises such as the jack knife. Doing an exercise I've never done before is so weird, and my body struggled, but by the second day I was already better at it. Emma talks about how you have to train your body:

EMMA

Our bodies are intelligent, you'll find that the first time you try a new exercise it seems nearly impossible, but the second time it seems easier; this is because your body is already adapting, seeking a path of least resistance to make something easier. This is why we have to keep moving forward, keep mixing things up! Never underestimate your body, it will try and defy you at every turn, you've just got to keep going!

I've been keeping my new clothes shopping to the minimum. I have 2 dresses I wear for work, but my casual trousers were too big, so I had to look for something new. It was great to go into Next and finding that all their size 18 trousers fitted with no need to breathe in to get the zip up. I knew these would soon get baggy, however, so instead I bought some cheaper ones which I'll be happier to dispose of in a couple of months.

Emma checked my measurements and it's been a great month: here is the monthly loss of cm, along with the total loss in the past 6 months:

MEASUREMENT REDUCTIONS

Bust	1cm
Biceps, right	3.9cm
Waist	6.7cm
Hips	4cm
Thigh, right	3cm
Calf, right	0.5cm

Over the past 6 months my overall drop in measurements is astounding.

Bust	From 136.5cm to 114cm. Loss of 22.5cm (nearly 9")
Biceps, right	From 36cm to 29cm. Loss of 6cm
Waist	From 133cm to 109cm. Loss of 24cm (nearly 9.5")
Hips	From 138.5cm to 114cm. Loss of 24.5cm (over 9.5")
Thigh, right	From 67cm to 59cm. Loss of 8cm
Calf, right	From 47.5cm to 45.5cm. Loss of 2cm

Saturday, 10 April 2010

I'm now on my 2nd programme with Emma, gosh it's hard, and I'm sweating a lot. She said that that's because I'm working on my inner core. We will go back to strength stuff next time. I'm now wearing sleeveless vests at the gym and today someone spoke to me and said that she had noticed how much I had improved over the months. I saw a large lady training with Adam (another PT) yesterday, probably about the size that I was at my biggest, I thought she had only just started but she has been working out with Adam since September. I asked Emma about her and she said that she doesn't focus on eating the right food and Adam had even taken her to the supermarket to show her what to buy. I think that's what has been making the difference with me, my inner motivation, you can't get your motivation from anyone else.

Today is carb day so I've had some bread and cheese and will have my champagne later.

Sunday, 11 April 2010

As I move into week 28, I can still make mistakes. I travelled to London today to do some consultancy. As usual in my hotel room there was a pack of biscuits and I ate them without thinking. What is even worse is that I also ate the complimentary biscuits on the train, given to me because I had a first class upgrade.

WEEK 28

Monday, 12 April 2010
Weight: 14 stone 12lbs
57lbs total loss

I got on the scales this morning and I've lost another pound this week making for a loss of 4 stone 1lbs in total since committing to a new way of eating and living back in October.

I was tempted to skip breakfast this morning but I knew this wouldn't be a good move so I ate my breakfast; a few strawberries rescued from the fruit salad, 2 hard boiled eggs and my lemon and ginger tea. I then walked for 45 minutes to the office. At work, lots of people commented on my weight loss and how good I look. Several asked me how I have done it. It sounds so easy when I tell others I eat less and exercise more, because this doesn't take the quality of my food or level of motivation into account.

Being away from home makes everything more tempting. I ate biscuits last night. I was able to resist today, but then I went to get some hot water and the late afternoon snacks were out, including some chocolate brownies. I couldn't resist and ate one without even thinking, without even tasting…I read the packet and saw they were 130 calories each. Not much but I hadn't really tasted this so I went ahead and ate another. Why oh why! It just goes to show that even after 28 weeks you can still get sidetracked.

I went out to dinner with some work colleagues, I managed to skip the wine and had satay sticks for a starter followed by a chicken and cashew nut stir-fry so I think that was good. Went back to the hotel, where I ate two biscuits. If they hadn't been in the room I wouldn't have eaten them. As Oscar Wilde said; 'I can resist anything except temptation'.

Tuesday, 13 April 2010

I woke up this morning and considered skipping breakfast, but knew that surely that wouldn't help me. Better to have my 2 boiled eggs again.

I've been thinking about what I ate yesterday. The 2 brownies were only 260 calories and when I add in the 2 biscuits that's about 400 calories. This shouldn't make much difference to my weight loss overall, it's possible to remain static for a day. I am going out for a meal tonight with Simon where I'll remain very focused, no alcohol again. Then, must stay super focused over the rest of the week.

I did a lot of walking yesterday, walking for 45 minutes in the morning and then walking up and down the stairs all day in the office. There were 2 flights between the floor I was on and the main office, 3 flights if I wanted to get a drink - I did as much walking as possible.

Wednesday, 14 April 2010

We had a meal out tonight, after 2 days away it was nice to take some time to chat with Simon. We had another Thai meal, I do like Thai food, I find it really tasty.

What I do need to do is to get back into the habit of eating every 3 hours, I was doing this and I'm not doing it consciously anymore. So this means eating at 8am, 10.30, 1pm, 3.30, 6pm and 8.30pm. I also need to continue with regular exercise.

WEEK 29

Monday, 19 April 2010
Weight: 14 stone 12 lb
57 lb total loss, no change

After 28 weeks, it's getting harder. Last night I had half a bottle of wine and a couple of oat biscuits and cheese. Not a huge amount of food but why? I think it is because I've been so busy with work that I needed time to unwind and alcohol always helps me do this.

I worked out very hard with Emma at the gym and sweated a lot! I managed to run (not jog!) for a whole minute, this really is awesome. Simon bought some crusty bread when we went shopping so I had some of that with my chicken and salad for lunch, I enjoyed it!

Saturday, 23 April 2010

I'm now at the end of week 29 and it is getting hard to eat so strictly. I have kept going for 6 months but this week I've had a glass of wine each evening plus 2 cream crackers with cheese in the evening. Last night I also ate some French bread with my meal, so not a huge amount of extra stuff, but I felt I needed to just eat a little more normally. I had a new workout with Emma yesterday and as I was learning a new programme so I didn't work out as hard as I can.

Emma and I discussed my exercise plan. I'm to alternate between a cardio and a weights session and on the days I don't go to the gym I am to go for a brisk 40 minute walk.

EXERCISE PLAN

You can read some examples of how my exercise has progressed in the appendix. The most important thing to remember with exercise is that you must continually strive to do more, if we can do 20 reps holding 3kg weights in each hand then next time try it with 4kg!

WEEK 30

Monday, 26 April 2010
Weight: 14 stone 10.5lbs
59.5lbs total loss

I might have eaten more than I wanted to yesterday but I have still lost 1.5lbs.

I did my hour of cardio with Emma today and it nearly killed me, it was such hard work, I have never had a session like this. Ben's approach was very different to Emma's and he was much more into strength training. Emma said it was important to do both, so I think I'll be aiming for 4 days a week of strength work and 2 days of cardio with a walk on the other day.

I'm going to Cheshire to see my family this weekend and if I can lose 2.5lbs by Saturday this will amount to a stone in 8 weeks! I'm pressuring myself to meet this target.

Tuesday, 27 April 2010

Not sure what was going on with me yesterday. I decided to try having porridge for breakfast. I've got lots of it in the cupboard and I didn't think it would hurt to eat it. I then had some pistachio nuts mid morning, that's not unusual, but rather than divide a bag into 4 so I was in control of my portions I started eating...and by the end of the evening the bag was gone. I had a client call at 12 so I had to rush and have a quick lunch as I was going shopping and then to the gym immediately afterwards. I don't think it is a good move to eat so quickly that I'm not really tasting my food. When I was shopping I bought Simon some wonderful stone-ground wholemeal bread, really nice stuff, but I was tempted by it! I did my workout, got home and had a slice of bread, butter and marmite, then another one. I'm now on a downwards carb roll!

For tea I had a small jacket potato with my turkey casserole, then in the evening I had two gin and tonics and a slice of toast with butter and marmite. I don't think this was a great day and if I want to lose 2.5lbs this week I need to stay über strong and focused till Saturday. On reflection, it was the morning carbs that lead to today's downfall.

'Winners never quit, quitters never win.'

Vince Lombardi

WEEK 31

Monday, 3 May 2010
Weight: 14 stone 10 lb
60 lb total loss

I only lost half a pound this week, but I ~~think~~ know I have been eating a little too much. I've had a glass of wine every night plus a couple of crackers with cheese. With Ben not around to tell me which food to eat I've lost my focus.

I visited family on Saturday and had a lovely time with my sister, she commented on how slim I looked, I think we are pretty much the same size on top but now I'm smaller around my hips. My nephews Oli and Julie both asked me how much I weighed and I told them.

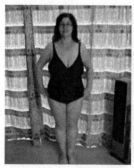 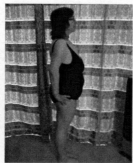 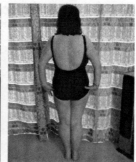

Previously I would have lied, I always used to knock a couple of stone off my weight.

I decided I needed some new clothes and we went to McKay's - I picked up a range of size 18 clothes and everything fitted! I've now got a wonderful dress to wear for our party and also a great turquoise top with a white wrap to wear over the top which looks very flattering. In Matalan I tried on 4 different pairs of size 18 trousers/shorts, all fitted me absolutely fine and I bought the leggings in a size 16 as the 18s were quite loose.

I probably had half a bottle of wine and some potatoes with my meal which was something of a wake up call. I have decided that I need to be fully focused from now on. This means no more wine for the next month apart from with my 'once a week' special meal.

Saturday, 8 May 2010

Simon and I went to our first festival of the season and this presented me with challenging decisions about what to eat. I've had one alcoholic drink each day, a pint of beer watching Iggy and the Stooges at All Tomorrows Parties and a glass of wine with my pizza tonight. On reflection I'd have done better with fish and chips rather than pizza as there was very little protein in it. I think I was seduced by the salad and I did have plenty but still think I should have opted for more protein. This hasn't really been much of a dance festival, I've spent more time standing around and watching the bands, so it's not been as energetic as some and as it is held at Butlin's Minehead everything was quite close together.

WEEK 32

Monday, 10 May 2010
Weight: 14 stone 6lbs
64lbs total loss

Woop, woop, I've lost 4 pounds. This is amazing and I'm very happy. I'd be kidding myself if I said I wasn't motivated more by these larger weight loss weeks.

Tuesday, 11 May 2010

I've been ill, despite taking all my vitamins. I felt cold on Saturday evening and woke up on Sunday morning with the most awful sore throat and I ached all over so we came home from the festival early. I went to bed on Sunday at 8pm and slept for 13 hours and still felt awful all Monday. Today I feel a bit better with less aches and shivers but I still have a sore throat. Because of this, I haven't done any exercise and yesterday I did eat a couple of slices of bread and cheese, being ill I really fancied this.

Sunday, 16 May 2010

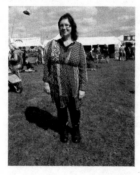 I've just got back from Bearded Theory Festival and I certainly wasn't one of the biggest women there this time. I remember when it was so very rare to find people that were bigger than me. I felt really good and looked good - look at the pictures.

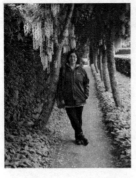
I also bought myself a new waterproof coat in size 18 instead of the usual size XXXL! I also bought a size 16 fleece, 2 x size 16 t-shirts and a mini skirt from Primark.

I wasn't able to stick to my usual diet and I do love Pie Minister but I managed to skip the mash and just have one each day. For breakfast we went to Wetherspoons where I had a bacon bap. I only ate the smaller half of the bread and also had yoghurt and fruit salad so this was a healthy breakfast overall in my eyes. I had falafels with lots of salad in a wholemeal pitta bread each day so I ate pretty well considering I was at a festival!

WEEK 33

Monday, 17 May 2010
Weight: 14 stone 3lbs
67lbs total loss

Yippee! I've lost 3lbs this week, making for a total of 8lbs in 5 weeks. Overall, I've now lost 67lbs since October which is only 3lbs short of 5 stone and my target is now to reach this by the end of the month at the latest. It has taken 10 and a half weeks to lose a stone, but it's still a stone lost at the end of the day. I think I've lost focus since Ben went off ill and have tried out different foods without his guidance. I think my weight loss has slowed because of this, however it has also been a time for me to 'tread water' and get refocused.

It's now been 32 weeks since I committed to getting fit and healthy and for a couple of weeks I tried out eating more, having a glass of wine at night, and the weight loss slowed. 6 months is a long time to follow a plan and it did me good to eat a little differently. I was still losing at least a pound a week whilst doing this. I'm currently still working out with my brilliant inspirational trainer, Emma.

From my very biggest I have lost well over 8 stone which amounts to 116lbs! If I lose another 40lbs I will literally be half the woman I was - will I do it? It will take time, but yes, I will!

Emma measured me today. I've lost about 2cm all over which is a very good result. What I'm most pleased with today is that I ordered 2 x size 16 denim skirts from Next and both fit me fine, I've not had to breathe in at all - I feel so happy.

MEASUREMENT REDUCTIONS

Bust	3cm
Biceps, right	2cm
Waist	1.7cm
Hips	2cm
Thigh, right	2cm
Calf, right	1cm

Did a killer work out with Emma after being measured. We concentrated on legs so I don't know why my arms hurt so much. Tomorrow it's cardio, then arms on Wednesday. I'm going to alternate floor work/weights and cardio - I want to lose 10lbs in 5 weeks and this is the way to make it happen!

Friday, 21 May 2010

I've been working out hard and also paid careful attention to what I eat. I haven't had many nuts except yesterday. I was being interviewed by Alvin Hall at BBC Radio Bristol (he flirted with me but I think he does it with every woman!) and needed to eat something as I drove to Gloucester for a meeting – had some nuts as I drove and a protein shake seemed like a reasonable lunch.

I am sweating a lot more at the gym. Emma says that the fitter I get the more I will sweat, plus I am doing more cardio. She has reminded me to do as much exercise as I can during the day and that this can include brisk walking.

Saturday, 22 May 2010

Full of a cold again. It can't be for lack of vitamins, maybe it's because I've been a bit stressed with work. After 2 weekends away at festivals it's been lovely to have a more relaxing time at home. Today I felt so rough and craved carbs. I normally wouldn't have given in as I don't have bread in the house but I had bought some tiger bread rolls for Simon so I ate a couple of those. I also had 2 portions of frozen yoghurt - Ben and Jerry's. This has fewer calories than the ice cream equivalent. I always used to eat straight from the tub but today I decided to measure out portions.

WEEK 34

Monday, 24 May 2010
Weight: 14 stone 1lbs
69lbs total loss

Another 2 pound loss and I'm very pleased! It was such a hot day today and yesterday we spent quite a bit of time making preparations for our summer party - less than 4 weeks to go now. Simon isn't feeling well and didn't want any food so I ended up snacking rather than having a proper meal.

I decided I was going to have a glass of wine on Sunday evening. I had planned to sit and watch TV, but I got focused on work and drank wine at my desk. Drinking while working meant I didn't savour it and I allowed Simon to top up my glass so I ended up drinking half a bottle of wine. I then ate a couple of crackers with cheese as my resolve weakened. This is not going to help me with my goal of losing 2lbs this week especially as I didn't go to the gym all weekend. I need to be much more focused if I want this to happen.

Wednesday, 26 May 2010

My eating hasn't gone well today and I think this is a good example of what happens when you are not well prepared. I had to go to the dentist first thing and thought there would have been time to shop before my appointment in the gym. My dentist was running late, the appointment took longer than I expected and I had to rush to the supermarket after the gym where I got caught up in queues. In the end I didn't get home till five past one. This should have been okay as my client wasn't due till 1.30pm but he was already waiting outside so I ended up eating 2 slices of ham as he had a coffee. I was hungry while we did our session and afterwards I ate a pitta bread with cheese, not a great move. For tea I ate falafels with a pitta bread and don't think this was a good move either. Finally I had a glass of wine - ummm, not great and felt very annoyed with myself.

DON'T BEAT YOURSELF UP

Things happen, we can't be perfect all the time. The worst thing to do is to let one set back set us up for many more. Even a day filled with poor choices is not going to cause long term problems if we start afresh the next day.

Friday, 28 May 2010

I think my period is going to start, despite the fact that I'm going through the menopause. I do get an occasional one, maybe that's why I've been hungry this week. Tonight I had a glass of wine, tea with a crusty roll and then strawberries, cream and malt bread. I think it is fine to have an evening like this every now and again, actually I do know it's not fine, I'm trying to convince myself. I did a good work out at the gym, worked on my arms and was pleased to be able to do stomach exercises – 3 sets of 20 crunchies and reverse crunchies!

Sunday, 30 May 2010

Yesterday I did an Alesha dance class at the gym plus we went to see Pendulum so I did lots of exercise as I love bouncing to drum n' bass. Today I had booked myself in for a second dance class and I was the only person who showed up so I ended up with a private lesson with Siobhan. Lots of people like classes and as I love music so much it was fun to do a dance class. I think I could have ate more for breakfast and lunch as this evening I was SO hungry. I ended up eating half a bag of nuts and a couple of oat cakes. Not a load of extra food but I don't normally eat so much at night.

WEEK 35

Monday, 31 May 2010
Weight: 14 stone 1lbs
69lbs total loss, no change

I got on the scales this morning and my weight remains the same. I probably should have expected this given what I ate on Wednesday. The past two weeks have been very good, I've been losing 2lbs each week and I think that is a lot to be losing now, I think a pound a week is more realistic. I still really want to get below 14 stone!

I did my legs workout with Emma and we discussed my diet. She said that if I don't lose weight this week she will get me doing more weights to shock my body. I wasn't sure whether or not to tell her that I ate half a vanilla cheese cake today. Whilst I loved it and ate it in 3 sittings, it is now sitting very heavy in my tummy and I know I really shouldn't have. When I did confess, Emma said 'I have no sympathy whatsoever!'

TELLING THE TRUTH

It's easy to lie to ourselves and to others. To pretend we didn't eat so much, to forget about the cake or sweets and misjudge the size of portions. What is the point of fooling ourselves, though? Being honest helps us to reflect on what happened and figure out what we can learn from it.

'Most people give up just when they're about to achieve success. They quit on the one yard line. They give up at the last minute of the game one foot from a winning touchdown.'

Ross Perot

Sunday, 6 June 2010

I've been at Sunrise Festival for a few days and although I've been walking about the site and dancing it's hard to keep to a plan when you are camping and have to eat from the traders. It hasn't been too bad - tofu curry, hog roast in a roll, not much alcohol, 2 pieces of cake, etc. so I expect my weight to remain the same. I read once that it is good to stabilise as it helps your body to get used to it's current weight and then when you start a strict eating regime again it kick starts the weight loss process once more. I will be on holiday this next week and we have our party coming up which means that I will plan to focus again from 21st June. I made some ginger cake for the party as I wanted to check out the recipe but it has been tempting and I've been eating some.

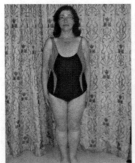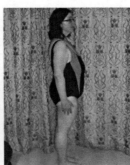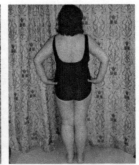

WEEK 36

Monday, 7 June 2010
Weight: 14 stone 3lbs
67lbs total loss, 2lb gain

On the scales today and I discovered that I'm 2 pounds heavier. It's all down to eating cake. I ate more than half a vanilla cheese cake, not good. If I want cake again I have to buy it when I have people over for a meal so my portion is limited. I also ate quite a bit of ginger cake I cooked to test a recipe the other day.

HOLIDAY DIETS

There's lots in magazines, newspapers and on day time TV about losing weight before the holidays. This happens every year around summer and then again in New Year but focusing on short term weight loss sets us up for yo-yo weight gain in the long run.

Thursday, 10 June 2010

On Tuesday we travelled up to Scotland. This meant spending 10 hours in a car so I hardly got any exercise aside from walking to the loo a few times at service stations. We had a bit of a walk around Nairn before dinner and then I had steak and chips with only minimal salad – I thought they would have provided much more. Just one glass of wine.

On Wednesday we walked around Nairn after a mediocre breakfast. The scrambled eggs were awful, no fruit so I had weetabix, then yoghurt then my eggs with a piece of dry toast. I thought we should do something active so we went to an outdoor centre, walked around the nature trail and then went to do the ropes course. Simon did it but I felt too nervous, I don't like heights, and had to come down. We needed lunch but it was hard to choose anything from the menu – nothing plain like chicken or salad so I had a half portion of tuna bake with salad. A half portion was big enough; goodness the portions are large here. I decided I didn't want another stodgy dinner at the hotel so I had a half pint of beer when we got back to the hotel and then ate some chicken and tomatoes in the room while I did some work.

PORTION CONTROL

Many of us eat bigger portions than we should. I used to eat large meals, sometimes even bigger than my husband's, but now I'm eating more mindfully and know that I don't need to eat everything on my plate. It does seem like a waste when restaurants serve such huge portions but just remember you aren't obliged to eat everything. At the pub, the night before Rockness, we could have shared a meal there was so much.

Friday, 11 June 2010

We're up in Scotland for the Rockness Festival. We took a boat trip on Loch Ness this morning and visited Urquhart Castle so did plenty of walking and I positively ran up the slopes and hills and steps. Lunch consisted of a set meal at the Indian so not a huge portion and we then did quite a lot of walking around the festival site. I did quite a bit of dancing and got to feel quite tired at the end. It was only afterwards that I remembered about all the walking earlier in the day in addition to all walking around the site. There wasn't much sitting down. We both noticed how many really large women there were. There was also another group who were quite slim apart from their enormous jelly belly; this is down to the food that people eat – too much fast food and sugar. For our evening meal Simon had a hog roast and I had a venison burger but left most of the bun.

Sunday, 13 June 2010

I did less walking around the festival site yesterday, but still managed plenty of dancing. We had a big breakfast which meant we didn't need lunch till later and I ate some chicken slices that I'd bought at the supermarket.

WEEK 37

Tuesday, 15 June 2010
Weight: 14 stone 6lbs
64lbs total loss, 3lb gain

Oh dear, I got on the scales this morning and I've now gained another 3 pounds. That's a 5lb gain in 2 weeks. Yesterday, the journey home was long (500 miles) and then there was the food. I had some muesli before we left the B&B, ate some wine gums on the journey, had a roast at a stop for lunch, then for tea I had 2 slices of cheese on toast. I followed this up with some duck spring rolls and a can of coke in the evening. Probably 2lb of this will go in a day or so, so I have only put on a pound, but even so ... during these past few weeks I have really deviated from my eating plan so from this moment onwards I will return to my original diet of low carb meals every 3 hours.

Food today:

- **Breakfast**: 2 boiled eggs.
- **Lunch**: salmon and salad, half a cucumber juiced.
- **Mid afternoon**: second piece of salmon and 8 cashew nuts.
- **Dinner**: haddock and salad, half cucumber juiced.
- **Supper**: chicken leg and strawberries.

I also went to the gym and did a workout which targeted the upper half of my body.

Friday, 18 June 2010

For 6 months I remained focused but after I changed trainer I lost some of this focus. It was hard to continue with such a strict eating regime so I added in some extra things. Eating things like oat cakes with cheese, having wine most evenings and reintroducing milk to my tea and drinking coffee again have all stifled my progress. I'm going to stay focused and go back to eating one carb meal every 5 days, just like I did before. I need to lose another 2 stone. Measurements today are not brilliant, but I am pleased to lose 2cm from my bust.

MEASUREMENT REDUCTIONS

Bust	2cm
Biceps, right	0.2cm
Waist	1cm
Hips	1cm
Thigh, right	0cm
Calf, right	1.5cm

Before I went to bed I tried on my new skirt from Next. I can fit into a size 14 short denim skirt and think I look great! Simon was very impressed with what I looked like and virtually threw me on the bed! He likes his slimmer wife.

Sunday, 20 June 2010

Yesterday was our party. It had taken a week of hard work and preparations but the day went well and everyone commented on how great I looked. I think it came as quite a shock to many people to see just how much weight I had lost. I ate cake and drank champagne but avoided the bread and cheese.

Today I felt so tired even though there was so much to do. I've also eaten more cake and cheese. I will freeze whatever cake is left at the end of the day. We do have a lot of cheese left but it will be eaten by Simon over the next few weeks.

STOP GRAZING

It's so easy to raid the fridge and eat standing up. It's far better to make the food look good on a plate and then sit down to eat. Eating mindfully will ensure we focus on our food instead of snacking.

WEEK 38

Monday, 21 June 2010
Weight: 14 stone 2lbs
68lbs total loss

I have been so focused this week. I think being so strict and doing some killer workouts at the gym has really shocked my body, resulting in a 4 pound loss this week. Only 32lbs to go and then I've lost 150lbs! There are 10 weeks until my birthday so if I could lose 20lbs by then it would be amazing! After that I would have just a stone to go. I have to be fully focused.

Another killer workout with Emma, we did strength training and I moved up to 105kg on the leg press.

Wednesday, 23 June 2010

My back is hurting more today. It's weird how the pain has moved from my left shoulder to my right shoulder. Emma said it's probably referred pain from a spasm in my trapezius, the muscle that runs along the back of my shoulders and down the mid of my back. I did my leg strength exercises but not the bar lifts as everything hurt and instead treated myself to a short massage. I've also been in the hot tub twice today. Earlier I bought some size 16 cropped jeans and they fit me, no problem at all, this is so brilliant! Tonight I had some left over wine and some cheese and crackers, I think I'm feeling sorry for myself because of my back!

Thursday, 24 June 2010

Got up very early to get in the queue for the new iPhone, so pleased I managed to get one. After that I went straight to the gym for a cardio session. The pain that is moving around the top of my back and neck is still present so I don't want to do strength exercises on my own.

Saturday, 26 June 2010

We went into Cheltenham shopping today, I'm much happier with how I look and now I don't mind looking at myself in shop windows.

We did a bit of shopping, I'm still wearing size 18 Sloggi maxi briefs which come up way past my waist so we went to M&S and I bought some pretty new shorts. I'll buy even nicer ones once I'm getting bras to match. I needed a new watch so we went and tried some on. I've previously had to wear a man's watch as my wrists were too big for a woman's. I feel so much joy wearing a woman's watch. I feel so much more feminine. This watch strap even needed to have a couple of links removed. I didn't go to the gym today or yesterday as we have been doing quite a bit of physical work sorting out the sheds, and doing all of this in the hot weather is heavy going enough!

Sunday, 27 June 2010

We had lunch at Simon's parents today. Mary had asked me what I wanted to eat so I was strict, didn't have cake but after watching everyone else I wish I had some. We went to the supermarket afterwards and I bought 2 slices of cheese cake and I ate both over the course of the evening, so I would have done better to simply have had a piece of cake at lunch time.

WEEK 39

Monday, 28 June 2010
Weight: 13 stone 13lbs
71lbs total loss

I have broken the 5 stone loss barrier in the past 38 weeks. This really is cause for celebration. Simon is so very proud of me, and I'm proud of me too! I've lost 8 and a half stone since my heaviest. I celebrated with strawberries and ice cream left over from our party. Umm not sure that was meant to happen but it was in the freezer. Big lesson, don't keep stuff at home that isn't good for your body. My back is hurting today and I'm not sure what has set it off. I was fine at the gym yesterday so it may have been caused by stretching as we took down our big festival tent from the party.

I tried on Simon's shorts today and they fit me! They are probably a closer fit than on him but they are a good fit around my bum, so they looked good! Don't think I'll fit in his skinny jeans just yet but I will try them on once I lose another stone.

I did strength exercises with Emma at the gym today. As we are both still a little concerned about my back we dropped the weights but upped the repetitions, we needed to do this so the muscles were still pushed to overload or they wouldn't adapt. There is always a way around a problem if you care to look.

This evening I was on the phone to my mum and walked around and around the garden as we spoke. I thought that this was an easy way to add in more exercise.

IT DOESN'T HAVE TO BE THE GYM

We need to perform physical activity during the week simply by doing everyday things we enjoy. It doesn't have to be a gym, we just need to think of physically demanding activities that will be pleasurable and enjoyable, such as playing with children or taking a dog for a walk. Walking when on the phone is a great way to add exercise into daily activities.

Tuesday, 29 June 2010

I felt hungry today and ate some ginger bread from the freezer, obviously not something I should do regularly. This led to me having a half bottle of wine. I don't do this every night so I think it is okay, but I'm left wondering why I did it.

I did cardio at the gym, spent 45 minutes working out very hard and I really did sweat a lot. Did a full set working out for 6 minutes at a time on 5 different pieces of equipment. I then did an extra 5 minutes work on the wave machine, bike and stepping machine. Finally, I did my inner thigh exercises, this time with 45kg of weights.

Wednesday, 30 June 2010

I heard on the radio this afternoon that lecturing people about their diet doesn't lead people to make changes. In fact Jamie Oliver's campaign for better school dinners has led to a drop in people staying for school dinners. How then, do we help people to make a change? One reason I wrote this book was so that people can read my story and see what is possible.

LOW FAT FOOD IS NOT THE ANSWER/ DON'T OVEREAT LOW FAT FOOD

Many people think that eating low fat food means they can eat more. Low fat means higher sugar, and high fructose corn syrup is not a healthy choice as it makes us crave carbs and sugar. A better choice is to have a small portion of the full fat option.

'To be successful you have to be willing to hit the gas when your body is begging you to hit the brakes.'
Leilana Munter, Race car driver

Thursday, 1 July 2010

I have eaten a bit more today than I had planned but I have also been doing extensive exercise. Anyway, stepped on the scales first thing and I'm 13 stone 11 and a half. I also think my period is due, so I'm happy with my weight and determined to eat strictly. When I type this it sounds like I'm going to starve myself but I'm not, I do eat lots of healthy foods.

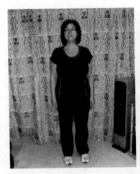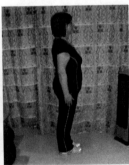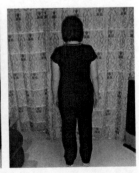

Yesterday I was hungry so I ate a portion of hazelnuts and also some oat cakes which is much better than cake or diet meals. My protein for tea was a venison burger and I had smoked mackerel for breakfast and lunch but somehow I don't think this was enough protein, think I'll cook a chicken today.

MEASURING PROGRESS

Weight loss is not linear, when the scales aren't changing we can also monitor progress by measuring

- how many times we have exercised
- how many steps we have walked
- how much water have we drunk
- how we feel

Friday, 2 July 2010

I still weigh 13 stone 11.5 pounds, but I have my period again. This is actually really interesting as I am in the throes of the menopause but with no symptoms as I eat healthily.

THE MENOPAUSE

The menopause is seen as a time where women experience many negative symptoms - hot flushes, night sweats, depression, headaches, insomnia, anxiety, weight gain. However, these symptoms are not common in India, China, rural Greece or Mayan cultures. Could they be attributed to cultural differences in the diet and level of activity? As I progress through the menopause I can say, hand on heart, that I have not had any negative symptoms. Luck or a positive side affect of my healthy eating?

I watched a TV programme - *Big meets Bigger*. One girl came back from America and had lost over a stone in 2 months, the other, barely anything. The first girl started running and is doing it for herself, the other wants to do it for her mum, it's hard to lose weight for other people.

Simon got himself fish and chips last night so I had a really small helping, having a taste was enough, I didn't want a lot but it was good to taste some and realise I could never eat a full portion again.

WEEK 40

Monday, 5 July 2010
Weight: 13 stone 11lbs
73lbs total loss

I've lost another 2lbs. I checked out my BMI index online and once I reach 12 stone 11 I'll just be overweight, no longer in the obese category and my BMI will be below 30 - can't wait to get there!

At my fattest, when I weighed 22.5 stone (315lbs), my BMI was 52.4. This was morbidly obese. In October 2009 I weighed 18 stone 13 (265lbs) and my BMI was 44.3, still morbidly obese. Today I weigh 193lbs and my BMI is 32.1 so I'm in Obesity class 1. When I reach 12 stone 11, (179lbs) my BMI will be 29.8 so I'll be merely overweight. To be in the normal weight band I need to weigh 149lbs (10 stone 09) which is 24.8 but this doesn't take into account of my muscle tone.

BMI

This is not a definitive, reliable indicator of health, fitness or obesity, but we can't use that as an excuse to ignore the findings. When we get strong and muscular like personal trainers, sports people (and me!) we may find our BMI indicates that we are overweight or even obese when we aren't.

Thursday, 8 July 2010

I have very prominent varicose veins and met with the consultant today to discuss treatment. I'm a bit worried that I'll be unable to do any hard exercise for up to two weeks but if this is the case then I can do lots before hand and then do lots of walking.

It said on the news today that children need to cut down on food as well as to do more exercise, stating the obvious. Far too many people think that because they've just played tennis or gone to the gym then they deserve that chocolate bar - no you don't!

MINDFUL EXERCISE

As always at the gym there are people walking on the treadmill chatting to their friends, sitting on the bike and texting, etc. This isn't the way to do it. We need to really focus on the exercise, focus on muscles working and growing and doing the exercise as best we can.

EMMA: It's called 'training intensity', without it you my as well be on the sofa.

Saturday, 10 July 2010

I've just realised I haven't had a sweat rash this year! Usually in the hot weather I get sweaty and need to use hydrocortisone cream under my boobs but this hasn't happened at all this year. My leg is hurting and it hasn't helped that I've been sitting in a car for 2 hours driving up north to see family. It was nice to see family however, and although my niece offered me lunch, I brought my own food with me - cherry tomatoes and chicken. I was offered Jaffa cakes and low fat bars, but they aren't things I should be eating and so I declined.

Sunday, 11 July 2010

Today has been very stressful although I don't think this book is the place to talk about it. I had a couple of hard boiled eggs and all should have been fine but I started to get cravings and I think it was the stress. The old me would have stopped at a service station for rolos, munchies and an aero. I resisted and I'm proud of myself for that.

MAKE THE CHOICE

We can choose to binge and enjoy eating the food now, but then feel guilty afterwards. Alternatively, we can choose to eat a healthy snack, wishing we were having the guilty treat only to later find that we feel virtuous about making the right choice.

WEEK 41

Monday, 12 July 2010
Weight: 13 stone 10lbs
74lbs total loss

I've lost another pound.

I felt tired this morning so my plans for the day changed. I worked till 11pm last night and then woke at 5.30am this morning. I thought I should try and sleep some more and didn't wake up until the alarm went off which was 5 minutes before being interviewed on the radio. I have a very busy day and I had planned to go and do cardio early, straight from my radio interview but my body isn't used to working out so early and I felt tired so I thought it best to leave it. I've been looking through my diary to see how I can fit it in and I haven't got a 2 hour gap, so instead I will do a number of 10 minute walks throughout the day. Not ideal but better than nothing. I'll just have to go to the gym on Sunday to make up for today.

On Facebook today I read 'XXX is rewarding her body with a blueberry muffin - well after putting it through the ordeal of 40 sit-ups 40 crossovers and 20 push ups I have to apologise somehow!'

Any gain from the exercise will be negated by the muffin!

WHEN WE CAN'T FIT IN A VISIT TO THE GYM

When we can't manage to find time to travel to the gym and do a workout then it is worth remembering that short, brisk walks still gets the body moving. Wearing a pedometer makes it really easy to add a few hundred steps here and there. It takes 100 steps to walk around my garden, and on occasion I've done it 10 times to add 1,000 steps into my day!

Today I have my size 16 jeans on. They are so big around the waist, I should probably have bought the size 14...still they only cost me £8. Simon keeps on telling me how good I look and keeps grabbing me, he really is proud of me now and much more interested in sex! I am as well, when I was so heavy I just wasn't interested, I didn't want him touching my body and his playful way of squeezing my rolls of fat was so hurtful, even though I never said so. Now I'm more assertive and I've told him I don't like him doing that. He's reassured me that he is amazed at how less there is and loves me even more.

Tuesday, 13 July 2010

Natalie and Evie came to see me today, it's lovely to get cuddles from my grand-daughter. I really enjoy seeing them each week. Today was so busy, answering questions on a Guardian Career Forum, meeting clients and setting up things with actors for my involvement in a film on graduate recruitment.

As Natalie was with me for lunch I bought some crusty bread rolls, oh dear this isn't good! I ate half a roll with my lunch and the other half with cheese in the afternoon. Our evening meal only contained a small amount of protein so I had the last roll with smoked salmon. I really shouldn't buy crusty/nice bread as it is as addictive to me as chocolate, I need to stop buying things in the house that I like so much as I don't think this does me any good.

CARBOHYDRATES

Any carbs not immediately used are stored in our liver or muscles in the form of glycogen. Once are glycogen stores are full, any extra is converted to fat.

IMPACT OF HIGH CARB MEALS

High carb meals and snacks can lead to a rise in blood glucose. Insulin is released and the body stores carbs as fat. As our blood sugar levels rise, we get cravings for more carbs, eat more carbs and get stuck in a vicious cycle. If we don't eat carbs we can feel shaky and moody. To break the cycle we must eliminate refined sugars and lower the amount of carbs we eat.

Wednesday, 14 July 2010

Yesterday was such a busy day! I didn't stop, working flat out with no spare time to just chill. Because of this, I ate more and had no time for exercise and to be honest felt I was running a bit ragged all day. Monday I'd worked till 23.20 and last night I worked till 23.15. I know this wasn't good as sleep is important but there was so much on. I'm feeling more in control today and with no clients I can relax tonight and plan on an evening walk to compensate for not doing any exercise yesterday. Actually, that's not true - I did dance around the living room with Evie as we watched Frank Turner on DVD.

A powerful day at the gym, I'm now leg pressing 115kg (up from 100kg on the 18th June), straight leg deadlift has increased from 12kg to 18kg and I'm still doing 15 repetitions. My Swiss ball ham curls are up from 15 reps to 24 reps. I'm also deadlifting a total of 37.5kg, up from 25kg; the smith incline press, with a 15kg bar, has increased slightly, and my shoulder press with the black bar has increased by 2.5kg. I've also increased the number of sets I do of this exercise from 3 to 4.

Today was measurements day. Looking at my results over 9 months it's remarkable, almost 12 inches lost from my waist, and not far short of this from bust and hips.

MEASUREMENT REDUCTIONS

Bust	1cm
Biceps, right	up by 1cm - this is a good thing!
Waist	2cm
Hips	1.3cm
Thigh, right	0.5cm
Calf, right	0.1cm

Over the past 9 months my overall drop in measurements are astounding.

Bust	From 136.5cm to 108.2cm. Loss of 28.3cm (over 11")
Biceps, right	From 36cm to 28.1cm. Loss of 7.9cm (over 3")
Waist	From 133cm to 103cm. Loss of 30cm (nearly 12")
Hips	From 138.5cm to 110.9cm. Loss of 27.6cm (nearly 11")
Thigh, right	From 67cm to 56.4cm. Loss of 10.6cm (over 4")
Calf, right	From 47.5cm to 42.6cm. Loss of 4.9cm (nearly 2")

Today I made a spur of the moment decision to change my hairstyle. It's looked pretty much the same for a few years now so I got it cut much shorter and I really think it looks great. I also had the urge to wear makeup and look nicely dressed for clients! Losing the weight is making me want to look more attractive overall.

I got on the scales this morning and I'm still 13 stone 11, obviously I need to make some adjustments, whatever I'm doing at the moment is what I need to do to maintain my weight but it is not enough to get the weight down. Looking back over this past week I realise that I didn't go to the gym on 2 days and I did have cheese and oat cakes on a couple of days so that is what will have led to my weight stalling.

Saturday, 17 July 2010

We left at lunchtime yesterday to go to 2000 Trees Festival. It's local so we'll travel to it each day. I noticed a lot of young girls had a lot of fat around their middle. I'm certain this is down to their diet which focuses on processed food, plus too much cider.

We visited Simon's parents to discuss the final preparations for their wedding anniversary party. I was wearing a belt and they were amazed at how much smaller my bust is and how small my waist is. It's been a bit hard getting used to compliments, I'm more used to people saying 'you look well' which I think is code for you've put on weight.

I got on the scales this morning and I haven't lost anything. I think this can be attributed to missing 2 gym appointments and eating too many oat cakes and too much cheese. I've got to make a concerted effort now.

It was good to stay at home and sleep last night rather than camp at the festival. I really do need a good nights sleep.

CLOTHES SIZES

I read in the paper about the actual sizes of a 16 dress size - bust is 39-41inches and hips are 41-44 inches. I thought I'd convert my cm measurements and it turns out that I'm above the standard size 16 but well within the range for my hips. I think I read elsewhere, however, that companies actually make clothes that are bigger than these measurements.

Sunday, 18 July 2010

I'm feeling tired today, walking around festivals these past couple of days has been quite tiring, but I have to go to the gym - I need to do some cardio.

WEEK 42

Monday, 19 July 2010
Weight: 13 stone 10lbs
74lbs total loss, no change

Today is a new day. I had half a bottle of wine on Saturday and Sunday plus some cake yesterday. I'm drifting, so it's no wonder I haven't lost any weight this week.

A hard (or good) workout, depending on how you define it – I was much stronger on all my exercises but it is so hard. Not sure I should be writing this down but I am having leaks when I squat, I'm going to have to improve my pelvic floor with specific exercises.

From today I'm going to log my food and document how I felt when I ate it and why I ate like I did:

09.00	2 hard boiled eggs; ate at my desk as I worked. Then fish oil and psyllium husk,
12.00	protein shake; straight after my workout
14.10	some nuts, I'd been to the hospital and hadn't taken any food with me, luckily I had a bag of almonds in the car,
15.30	1 roll mop herring and some tomatoes; just got home from hospital and shopping and was hungry. I also had a diet ginger beer,
18.15	chicken and vegetable stew; if I had been at home I'd have had a 2nd half bowl but had to leave for the station,
19.30	banana and apple on the train,

22.00	6 almonds, found a few in a bag in my handbag, some tomatoes, banana. Think I should have brought some cold chicken. I certainly don't feel stuffed and if I was at home may well have picked at oat cakes and even had some cheese. I have to STOP eating oat cakes and definitely cheese. I will meet my objective! In fact 13 stone 3 is my first goal, I should be aiming for 12 stone 13

Alongside logging my food I need to up my exercise so I'm going to the gym 5 times a week. I also needed to add in more exercises – a walk to the railway line each day (3 mile round trip) plus squats every 30 minutes in my office.

Tuesday, 20 July 2010

New day, new start. I'm working in London today so I brought 2 boiled eggs with me for breakfast. I then walked to the office which was well over a mile away. I should have worn my pedometer. Stopped off at the local Sainsbury's and bought some cooked chicken, tomatoes and blueberries for later.

When I got to the building the doorman was very complimentary and said I looked about 20 – bless him! Lots of other assessors commented on how I look. I took the compliments to heart because I know I look good in my bright dress and heels!

My food intake today has been a bit repetitive, eating chicken and tomatoes all day, but that's what happens when you have to buy food whilst you're away. I am very pleased that I've said no to biscuits all day. It would be so easy to eat a packet or three (four?) but will that get me closer to my goal? No!

I'm going to go back to eating like I ate when I was training with Ben. I do miss working out with him and know that I'd be at least half a stone if not a stone lighter if I had been able to carry on with him. I can't allow myself to second guess what might have been however, it all comes down to what I do next.

Time to really focus, not time to give in. I remember years ago, when I was in my early 20s, I lost 5 and a half stone in 6 months, I never cheated, never gave in. But after 6 months this time I have, and that's been okay; cheating every now and again has only slowed things down. I don't want things to move slowly, however, I want to reach my goals now!

I really think that keeping a food log and planning when I will eat and what I will eat is a good move. I need to make sure that I eat 6 small meals every day. This is what I used to do with Ben – plan so I know what and when, and to make sure to eat 6 small meals. and I know this produces results so why did I stop?

Oh dear, I've just eaten a small chocolate brownie, I forgot they have snacks in the assessor's room and I had eaten it before I thought about what I was doing! Still, I did only have the one and it only took me three bites to get through it but I still shouldn't have. No point in beating myself up now though, what's done is done.

It will be nearly 10pm by the time I get home. I had yet more chicken and tomatoes but I'm getting sick of these so I didn't eat so much. Had a coffee and a small bag of mixed nuts, it really was a small bag as it was complementary.

I think if I add up the calories from everything I consumed today the total will still be quite low. I also got quite a bit of walking in. I'll be glad to get home and I should manage to clear my desk of reports by lunchtime although being at home I have the distractions of emails.

Just got home and had a second bag of nuts - each bag weighs 27gms. 100gms of nuts has 614 calories which means that I consumed 332 calories between the two bags.

Simon had put a bottle of wine in the fridge but I told him, in no uncertain terms,to put it away, we weren't going to have it!

Wednesday, 21 July 2010

Woop, woop, got on the scales this morning and I weighed in at 13 stone 8 pounds. A 2lb loss! I really am going to stay focused from now on.

09.15	smoked mackerel. Been really busy, forgot to eat till now.
12.00	protein powder after the gym.
14.00	chicken and tomatoes and an apple.
16.00	nectarine.
18.00	sword fish and salad.
21.00	strawberries.
23.00	protein shake.

A very hard workout with Emma as usual. I stayed very focused today. I had a lovely chat with my friend Carol and it was good to talk instead of working. When I told her how much I ate she was quite amazed. I do eat a lot of food, but it's all good food.

Thursday, 22 July 2010

09.00	smoked mackerel.
10.30	protein shake.

13.00	roll mop and tomatoes plus 25 grams of cashews.
16.00	piece of chicken.
19.00	2 pieces of sea bass and big plate of salad.
20.00	apple.

I went to the gym for a cardio session. There, I got chatting to some of the fitness instructors. They were amazed to discover that I've lost 125lbs (nearly 57kg). I was wearing my denim skirt and tight fitting T-shirt, Adam said I looked good in a skirt and said my husband must be getting frisky - he is.

I have so much energy! I had my facial today and Jo, my beautician, said I have a very firm bum! I still have flab on my inner thighs, but my exercise regime will continue to tackle that!

Saturday, 24 July 2010

I'm hosting my parent in laws' 60th wedding anniversary party in our garden tomorrow so Simon and I have been really busy getting everything ready. We did have time to eat and I made some pork casserole which we had with some veggies, but I don't think I had enough protein. I was so busy I didn't have time to relax and read the paper. Not a good thing. It really is important to relax and remain calm to stop stress from affecting my health.

Sunday, 25 July 2010

We were up really early today to get everything ready, I wanted to make it as spectacular as a wedding reception and it really did look beautiful. I wasn't sure what to wear and opted for my new leggings and heels, I'm looking good! I haven't worn heels for ages! I put them on at 9.30am and didn't take them off till 5.30pm, as I weigh less I can cope with the pressure they put on my feet for longer. So many people commented on how great I looked and Simon was very proud.

WEEK 43

Monday, 26 July 2010
Weight: 13 stone 5lbs
79lbs total loss

OMG, I got on the scales this morning and I weigh 13 stone 05, that's a 5lb loss this week! It just goes to show what you can do when you focus! This week I really have done everything right. I'm eating every 3 hours again, logging all my food and not eating carbs. I know this approach works so why did I go off track? It is hard to comply month after month and it is nice to drink wine, eat cake etc ... I wasn't over doing it, and my weight remained pretty stable, so at least I know what I need to do when the time comes to maintain my weight. Right now though, I still have 17lbs to shift to reach the magic '10 stone lost' milestone.

Wednesday, 28 July 2010

I'm in London on a consultancy assignment. For breakfast I had tinned grapefruit and 2 boiled eggs then I walked for well over an hour from the hotel near Paddington station to Westminster. I brought my own lunch so had chicken and tomatoes and then I went and had 2 small chocolate brownies, I know I know...I should have resisted but I'm feeling tired and they were there. But that was all I had.

Yesterday I started a new programme at the gym. We did supersets, doing exercises in sets of 2 rather than 3. It's always challenging to do new things for the first time and doing squats with 12kg weights in each hand was very hard going.

Thursday, 29 July 2010

I had hoped to go to the gym for some cardio today but I realised it was going to be too much for me. I had a desk full of work and I had to get a train to Salisbury for filming. I'm involved with a video on graduate recruitment. The Director was running late so I spent almost 2 hours talking with his wife, she is very focused on eating healthy food so we swapped food stories and I talked about how much I had lost. I was so pleased to have lost weight in time for the filming and I was also glad that I was wearing a colourful dress; the other two people I saw on video were in dark suits. The dress I wore for filming actually seems a little loose, so I wonder how long it will be before I get rid of that?

Hazel gave me a lovely salad for lunch with a nice dressing. I really ought to create a nice salad dressing myself rather than have it plain like I do, but anything is better than the bottled stuff.

Friday, 30 July 2010

It was a stretching day at the gym. I really worked as hard as I could but as I'm learning new exercises I'm not sweating as much. There were 2 young guys there, one with his shorts really low showing off his underpants - I asked him why he wore them like that, Emma was amazed I asked but I wanted to know. (He said they were more comfortable). I'm becoming fearless in what I say to other people and I am so much more confident. I used to be worried that people would retort and mention my size but I'm just normal looking now. Soon I will look fantastic!

A few weeks ago I bought some new jogging trousers from Next in a size 16, tried them on yesterday morning and they fitted fine but after my trip to the gym I realised I should have bought the 14s as they are already baggy! I think I will stay in my baggy clothes until I can buy size 12s, it's getting expensive buying new clothes that only fit for a few weeks.

I got some new bras and I'm now a 36G, but next time I'll be a 34. My bras are now prettier, with thinner straps and only 2 hooks at the back. I went through my wardrobe again and pulled out loads more clothes to take to the charity shop – there are now very few left in my cupboard.

PRETTY BRAS

I think at my biggest I was a 48HH, I could have been bigger. You can't buy a pretty bra in that size. As I dropped through the sizes I have had so many functional bras, but getting to a size where I could buy bras from Bravissimo was a brilliant milestone, I can now buy matching sets.

My client yesterday told me that I had a very muscular build, I like that, I want to be seen as strong!

'There is no such thing as unrealistic goals, only unrealistic time frames.'

Unknown

WEEK 44

Monday, 2 August 2010
Weight: 13 stone 3 lb
81lb total loss

I'm feeling great. On the scales and I've lost another 2lbs, that means I now weigh 13 stone 3 pounds, almost a stone off since our solstice party and on track for another 8lbs off by my birthday, so I could be a stone and a half lighter and close to 12 stone 07.

I posted on Facebook: 'Yes! lost another 2lbs - total loss since October is 80lbs, also doing new strength exercises including barbell back squat with 30kg, split squats with foot elevated and 8kg in each hand and bent over rows with 27.5kg'.

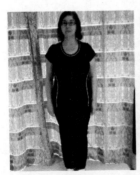 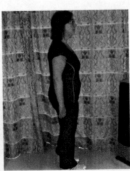 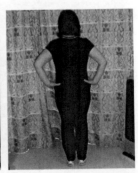

ALL CALORIES ARE NOT THE SAME

It is important to eat highly nutritious food. When we focus on calorie counting we can make poor food choices. We can decide to have a biscuit rather than an apple or a chocolate bar rather than a chicken salad. The same number of calories but some are healthy choices and others contain little of nutritional value.

As I eat breakfast I consciously eat slowly, savouring all my food, so I get more nutrients and feel sated quicker. I know when I was very fat I used to eat very quickly, I think I thought that the calories didn't count if I ate quickly.

Wednesday, 4 August 2010

Today the gym was hard work. I did what I normally do but only managed 3 of my 3rd superset. Emma and I observed one of the other gym members, he looked at one of the machines, made a phone call, started eating, did 3 reps, ate some more, 4 reps, or maybe 3 then sat down. Did he really think he was working hard? So many people think they are working out hard, they may put in the time but their level of effort is low.

WEEK 45

Monday, 9 August 2010
Weight: 13 stone 4lbs
80lbs total loss, 1lb gain

Oops! Got on the scales this morning and I've put on a pound! I think this is because I have eaten more than I should. Crackers and pate yesterday, half bottle of wine, slice of cheesecake and cheese and biscuits plus I only slept just over 4 hours last night. I was so busy, worked late, couldn't get to sleep then I was awake just before 5.15am. I also didn't get to the gym yesterday, didn't do any exercise at all, not even a walk to the bottom of the road.

My car was at the garage for a service today so I did a very brisk two mile walk to collect it. Another messy day. I had to go into Cheltenham for a dental x-ray and do some phone rehearsals with actors. Amidst all of this there was the lure of crusty bread so I ended up having 3 slices with cheese. I knew this wasn't a good move but I wanted it and saw it as a treat. Tonight I tried on Simons' Weird Fish fleece and it fits me well, not tight at all, so I now fit in his clothes. I know that when I lose another stone I'll be a size smaller still.

Thursday, 12 August 2010

It's been such a busy week, knowing I was going to be filming for a couple of days meant that I had to get straight with my work before I went and I felt really stressed out. It's so hard being careful about what you eat when you don't have time to relax. On Monday I had less than 15 minutes to eat before I found myself back at work talking to actors. Eating my salmon salad as quickly as possible isn't what I had in mind when I promised to savour my meals! It's no wonder that in the evening I had 3 cans of diet ginger beer plus some ginger cake, not good - I need to take myself in hand.

On Monday I saw Emma at the gym, it was a good workout but I didn't sweat as much, the weather isn't as hot and I never sweat as much doing strength exercises as I do with cardio. I had planned to go for an early morning cardio session on Tuesday but since I was heading off to London this proved unrealistic, I had so much work to do.

On the train I carried rather than pulled my suitcase and found it easy to put it in the overhead rack. It's brilliant how I can now walk down the standard class aisle without having to turn sideways. Close to me on the train was a larger lady who walked down sideways and struggled to get in and out of her seat - no struggle for me anymore! I found myself noticing her as she was sat on the other side, just in front of me so I had a good view, first she ate a large roll, then a huge bar of chocolate, then started on a bag of sweets...that was me a few years ago, but not now.

I ate well whilst away, just had a couple of biscuits including one chocolate one. I had no desire to binge, so I really have broken the habit with that. This morning I was on the radio, I usually wake up at 6.00am so didn't see a need to put the alarm on but I overslept, not ideal but think I carried it off okay!

No time this morning to go to the gym, but I knew I had to go so went in the afternoon and did a 30 minute cardio session. I feel quite stressed and even the exercise didn't help. I am looking forward to the 2 weeks without work that are coming up to get my stress levels down.

MEASUREMENT REDUCTIONS

Bust	3.5cm
Biceps, right	1.7cm increase!*
Waist	9.5cm
Hips	1.5cm
Thigh, right	1.5cm
Calf, right	1.5cm

* This is a good thing, it means I'm gaining a bicep muscle.

This evening we went round to see my daughter in law as it is her birthday, it was a nice evening, we met her parents who were very surprised at how much weight I had lost. They haven't seen me for ages.

WEEK 46

Monday, 16 August 2010
Weight: 13 stone 5 lb
79lb total loss, 1lb gain

My weight has gone up by another pound. I know I have been eating more, I found Simon's crusty bread and made myself a big cheese door stopper sandwich. The difference is that now I really enjoy it whereas in the past I'd have eaten it very quickly - not sure where I got the idea from that if you wolf something down it doesn't count!

On Saturday I had dental treatment - the first of a three stage dental implant plan. I know I can't eat anything for at least a week, well I can eat, but only soft stuff. The first day I was in quite a bit of pain, same on Sunday, and I'm not sure why but I was really hungry. Maybe it was because I didn't have anything to chew? I was told that ice-cream would be good for me, well I know how fattening that can be so instead I chose Ben and Jerry's frozen yoghurt. I got through a tub in just over a day, and I'm working my way through the second tub, but it does have a lovely numbing effect and frozen yoghurt contains half the calories of ice-cream.

Yesterday and so far today I've felt less hungry, more like I do normally, but I'm not doing much exercise so I must be careful not to eat too much. I think my carb intake has gone up as I'm eating mashed bananas which are easy to eat but are basically full of carbs. I'm even going to have shepherd's pie tonight and I loathe mince but everything I eat has to be soft so I have no choice really.

Because of my dental treatment I'm taking 2 weeks off from clients. Not having clients and resting more will be good for me. I think it's what my body needs as I have been working so hard.

Wednesday, 18 August 2010

TIP: When you make excuses, the only person you fool is yourself.

I thought about this as I waited to see Emma and I heard another gym member making excuses to her PT. The reason I'm doing so well is that I stay focused and keep moving slowly towards my goal and if I do something that isn't helping such as have a big thick cheese sandwich or more than one slice of cheese cake I don't then think, 'this is it I might as well give up', I just get back on the horse.

Today with Emma I did exercises on the mats rather than using the heavy weights. It was really interesting to do exercises that I haven't done for months - like press ups - I'm so much stronger and my inner core is stronger thanks to all my squats. I've had to do a different style of exercise as using heavy weights increases heart rate and therefore blood pressure which could put more pressure on my mouth and make my head ache.

Thursday, 19 August 2010

I enjoyed spending time away from work and I'm using this opportunity to do lots of tidying up around the house. I've gone through my clothes again and have pulled out even more clothes that are too big. Sizes are so strange, I had some men's size 34 waist Levis that are now falling off me but I have also got some size 34 jeans from Primark and these are a snug fit, and they look good! I've bought a size 16 white shirt from M&S which fits well, but another white shirt, admittedly a loose fit, was too big even thought it was a size 12. I also bought two other tops in a size 14, both have some stretch and this makes them a good fit.

As I've become too small for my old clothes I've enjoyed giving them away. Rather than keep them in the loft for when I put the weight back on I've been giving them away through Freecycle as plenty of other people had need of them. Each time I handed them over I told my story, and hope to have encouraged others to believe that they could do it too!

Friday, 20 August 2010

I did a good workout with Emma and met a friend in the afternoon. We had to queue for lunch in M&S and when I was out shopping I got very tired. I was also feeling more pain in my teeth. I'm not sure if it was getting tired that set it off but I knew I needed to get home. I then realised the pain was much worse so I called the dentist who removed two stitches and gave me more antibiotics.

Sunday, 22 August 2010

Two days at V Festival meant lots of walking and casual exercise. It rained yesterday but today was hot. I hadn't expected this so have ended up with burnt shoulders. It was hard to know what to eat but settled for curry and rice because it was soft, although my teeth were feeling much better by this point.

I bought a t-shirt, the L was a size 12, but I still bought it and I know it will fit me fine in a couple of months. I told the girl who served me that I'd lost 9 and a half stone, she asked me how I'd managed to do that but the more important question is how was I able to put on so much weight in the first place?

> TIP: 'Wanting to be thin is not enough, you also need to take action and continually work towards a goal.'

On Saturday I was sat on the ground watching a band with my knees bent and a man came up to me and said 'nice knees', I could have kissed him. I told Simon who agreed that I have nice knees and he kissed me.

On Sunday as we were stood watching The Coral a man walked by and said 'nice tits'! Very forward of him but the good thing is that I'm now looking good and will look even better soon!

WEEK 47

Monday, 23 August 2010
Weight: 13 stone 4lbs
80lbs total loss

I've lost a pound and I'm glad to be losing weight again.

Tuesday, 24 August 2010

I'm really not sure why I had an eating day yesterday; maybe it was because I bought some tiger bread rolls that called out to me - I had one for lunch and one in the evening. Yesterday I also missed a meal and just had a protein shake for breakfast as we had travelled back from V Festival.

Yesterday I had treatment on my leg. I had opted for the foam treatment for my varicose veins rather than surgery. This treatment was nowhere near as bad as the dental treatment but as the foam was injected it did feel sore, the consultant said it was bruising my leg. The nurse wrapped my leg in bandages and then put a support stocking over the top. I have to keep all of these on till Saturday, which means no shower. After this it's the compression stocking for another week.

Sunday, 29 August 2010

Today was my birthday and I had the best birthday ever! In the morning I made a casserole for 30 people but the main lunch was delivered from Waitrose. I set everything up in the garden - just like we did for Simon's parents' 60th wedding anniversary - with wine glasses and proper cutlery. We had a lovely lunch and then there was time to chill and chat in the afternoon before afternoon tea. Friends came round for the evening and we had Jon Gomm, an amazing guitarist, as our entertainment. I didn't eat a lot today, I never do at our parties, but I enjoyed having some champagne.

WEEK 48

Monday, 30 August 2010
Weight: 13 stone 0lbs
84lbs total loss

Another week where I dropped 4 pounds. What I find really odd is that the biggest losses don't always come during the weeks when I've eaten the least. Time to get the house and garden back to normal. This always means a busy day but we had my nephew, Oliver, helping which was good. We did take things easier than usual and found some time to chill out.

Tuesday, 31 August 2010

First day back at work and I had so many enquiries and emails to work through. I decided not to go to the gym but looking back on today I haven't done much exercise and I've eaten a slice of cake and some profiteroles. This is the worst thing about throwing a party, having the leftover food. Thinking about what else I ate today it wasn't too bad - 2 boiled eggs, a roll mop and tomatoes for lunch then ham salad with a small jacket potato for tea and 2 malted milk biscuits, plus a glass of wine. However, I haven't been having my cucumber juice.

'[Do not] assume it is impossible because you find it hard.
Recognise that if it's humanly possible then you can do it too.'
Marcus Aurelius, Roman Emperor

Friday, 3 September 2010

Just weighed myself this morning and I'm still at 13 stone, I'm pleasantly surprised because I thought my weight may have shot up a couple of pounds. With my nephew staying we've been eating and drinking more and we've also been finishing off the food from our party. I haven't been doing as much exercise as usual before but that's partly down to my leg treatment.

Yesterday I felt like I should eat less as I ate quite a lot on Wednesday but skipping a meal is never a great idea. Yesterday my food intake was as follows:

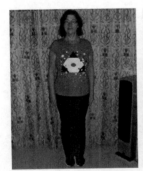 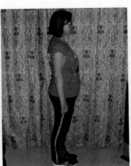 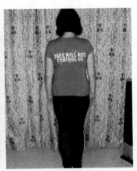

- **Breakfast**: nothing, wasn't hungry.
- **Mid morning**: chicken and veggies.
- **Lunch**: small piece of mackerel and cucumber juice.
- **Mid afternoon**: frozen yoghurt.
- **Dinner**: ribs of beef and roasted veggies, cooked in coconut oil, 1 small potato; large glass of wine, frozen yoghurt.
- **Supper**: ginger cake.

Today is a new day so I will get back to normal and tonight Oli and Simon will go out for a meal as I have a client and I will be stricter with my food intake.

Sunday, 5 September 2010

Spent yesterday in Manchester at the Muse gig where I burnt plenty of calories jumping about as they played. We had room only at the hotel and I hadn't planned for breakfast so:

- **Breakfast**: half a panini at Starbucks on the motorway.
- **Mid morning**: smoked mackerel and tomatoes.
- **Lunch**: ribs of beef, cauliflower cheese and a jacket potato.
- **Mid afternoon**: ginger cake and clotted cream.
- **Dinner**: 2 boiled eggs and 1/2 bottle of wine.
- **Supper**: ginger cake and clotted cream.

I was using up the cream from my party but did I really need to eat it? Overall, not a great food day but it's been a busy and stressful week. I loved having Oli staying but I have been eating more with him around and we have also had the stress of a death in the family.

Sometimes you just need to eat and drink, but where I would previously wolf my food down, I now savour every mouthful, most of the time!

WEEK 49

Monday, 6 September 2010
Weight: 12 stone 13lbs
85lbs total loss

I got on the scales this morning and I've lost another 1lb so I now weigh 12 stone 13. I've broken through the 13 stone barrier. Being in the 12 stone range seems normal. Yesterday was such a good eating and exercise day:

- **Breakfast**: ham and tomatoes
- **Mid morning**: nuts
- **Lunch**: ham and tomatoes (sell by date so wanted to finish off)
- **Mid afternoon**: 6 almonds
- **Dinner**: brisket and veggies
- **Supper**: apple

Today was good, too:

- **Breakfast**: scrambled eggs and tomatoes.
- **Mid morning**: protein shake.
- **Lunch**: roll mop and salad for lunch.
- **Mid afternoon**: 6 almonds and an apple.
- **Dinner**: brisket and veggies.
- **Supper**: apple.

I was working with a client today who told me about some special scales which also measure body fat, think I may order these. I continue to talk about my weight loss and eating and exercise plan with people I meet, it really helps me to stick with it. I'm come so far on this journey that there is now no going back.

Friday, 10 September 2010

This morning I'm tired and didn't go to the gym. I had some cheese and crackers, not great. I think when you get tired you crave carbs and high fat foods.

EMMA

When you haven't eaten enough it's like running a car without petrol, it won't work properly but unlike a car our bodies won't grind to a halt because they are intelligent and instead they will make us crave the nutrients they need, in this case the carbs in the crackers (for energy) and the protein and fat in cheese – never miss meals or you'll suffer the consequences!

WEEK 50

Monday, 13 September 2010
Weight: 12 stone 10lbs
88lbs total loss

Another 3 pound weight loss. Today I started a new programme at the gym and it was very tough. A focus on legs and doing stuff that REALLY

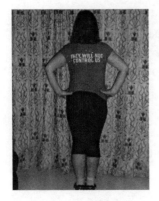

stretched me. We did measurements today, I've lost about 1cm all over. Simon also took photos and I think I look very good in my new Muse T Shirt. I'm most proud of the changes to my bicep measurements because I know my flab is firming up.

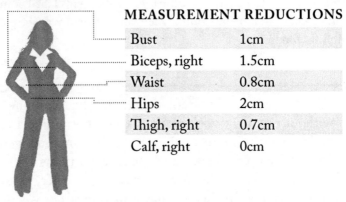

MEASUREMENT REDUCTIONS

Bust	1cm
Biceps, right	1.5cm
Waist	0.8cm
Hips	2cm
Thigh, right	0.7cm
Calf, right	0cm

The 3 pound loss is all the more welcome considering the fact that I also ate some carbs and drank alcohol this weekend, I think this behaviour ties in with being tired, it's not good to be tired. Yesterday in the Sunday paper I was surprised to read *'Obesity expert urges NHS to offer 1m Britons gastric bypass'*. Nick Finer, professor of obesity, has suggested that the best way for the NHS to tackle the health impact of the obesity epidemic is to set up a national network of fat clinics to provide gastric bypass surgery, he says the weight loss is permanent. However, there are many stories of people who lose the weight via this method but still put it back on as they haven't addressed the underlying psychological reasons. In addition, all these people will also want to have excess skin removed. Surgery is not the only way. Hopefully this book will show you how you can do it yourself.

SAGGY SKIN

People often wonder where all the skin goes when you lose a lot of weight. After a gastric band, people need further surgery to cut away excess skin,. The older we are the harder it is for our skin to remain elastic. After losing over 10 stone, my skin is pretty firm and I'm happy to be seen with bare arms, a real benefit of lifting weights whilst losing weight.

EMMA

Diet alone, or a gastric bypass/band, will get rid of visceral fat (fat that's 'within' the body), but it won't get rid of subcutaneous fat (fat that sits below the skin); only exercise and diet can do this and by targeting subcutaneous fat our skin is given the chance to 'shrink' back with us! So get lifting those weights and keep that body toned and honed!!

I didn't go to the gym on Saturday, I really was busy with shopping and tidying up so think I was quite active regardless.

I had some chocolate today, why? Because it was in the house, kit kats that I bought for Oliver, I should have given them to him to take away.

Tuesday, 14 September 2010

Today I had my teeth whitened. I had no idea I was going to be in so much pain! It has set my teeth on edge, I've also got to be very careful about what I eat and drink over the next 2 days, and once again I've got to eat soft food.

Wednesday, 15 September 2010

I have been so hungry today. Whilst shopping, I bought some soft bread and ate 3 slices of bread and jam. Staying focused is hard when I can't eat solid food and I have to be careful about not having anything that might stain my teeth. I was also getting a bit stressed; this was partly to do with choosing our holiday which should be a pleasant experience but I found myself getting bogged down in the research. I ended up having a couple of gin and tonics this evening.

Thursday, 16 September 2010

Went for a check up with my consultant this morning to check on my varicose vein treatment. Today I ate better but I was hungry again this evening so I had 3 oat cakes. I'm now having to drink coffee through a straw to stop my teeth from getting stained. I gave up coffee for 8 months but I started drinking it again in the summer, just a couple of mugs of fresh coffee each day.

Saturday, 18 September 2010

Shopping first thing, then the gym where I did my cardio and abdominal exercises again, a good start to the day. I know I'm going to eat more today and tomorrow as my mum and Roger are staying. Emma gave me a good tip; just eat half. Only one glass of wine and only half of my pudding. It was good to see my mum, she is amazed at her ever shrinking daughter and I do look good in my shorts! She tried on my size 14 fairisle dress, it's too big for her so she'll buy the size 12, and I said I'll have it from her once she gets fed up of it :).

WHEN YOU WANT PUDDING

Share with someone or just eat 3 bites. Better to leave it on your plate than regret it the next day.

WEEK 51

Monday, 20 September 2010
Weight: 12 stone 13lbs
85lbs total loss, 3lb gain

TIP: A few bad choices can destroy progress - you must focus on your goal.

Well what's going on? I've gone up again. Yes I've eaten some bread and cheese and drunk some gin and tonics...I know its not a real increase but even so it's bringing me down. The old me would have taken this as an excuse to eat chocolate. I do know that over the past week I've eaten 4 kit kats, I found them in a cupboard and it would have been better to throw them away. I spoke with Emma at the gym, she said it will be fluid retention, but I also haven't had as much cucumber as I'm scared of staining my teeth.

EMMA

The body **cannot** synthesise 'bad foods' into fat overnight, it takes at least two weeks so the only explanation is excess fluid retention due to the processed carbs in bread and **alcohol**! For each molecule of carb ingested between 1 and 2 molecules of water attach to them so they can be processed... more bad carbs = more water!

I had a lovely day with my mum, Roger and Simon's parents yesterday. It was relaxing and later we got in the hot tub. We cleared all 3 bottles of wine and I've told Simon that until I get to 11 stone 11 (150lb loss) I'll not drink any more wine, I have to reach my goal!

Thursday, 23 September 2010

Last week I ate more bread because my teeth were sensitive from the laser whitening. I don't understand how my weight could have increased by 3lbs in a week. I thought that I'd quickly lose it, that it was probably going to be glycogen/water but I got on the scales today and I've only lost 2lb. I know I ate more over the weekend with having my mum to stay. This week I've been much stricter and I had a very good work out with Emma on Monday and again on Wednesday.

THE CLOSER TO THE GOAL, THE HARDER IT GETS

I've put on weight and I'm disappointed, but I won't give in. We all have these challenges. I've just got to keep focused. It was much easier to lose weight when I was heavier as it took more calories to simply keep me alive!

I listened to a doctor on the radio who said that most of the people who come to see her are not interested in talking about healthy eating or exercise, they just want a pill to make them thin. Life isn't easy however and it takes a lot of excess food to put weight on. Accordingly, it takes a lot of time and effort to lose it as I'm showing.

There are just over 2 weeks till my one year weight loss anniversary and I want to be at 12 stone 6 or 7 by then so I'll have lost 10 stone and another 10 pounds to go by Christmas. It's quite depressing as my teeth whitening has set me back, and I don't feel like going to the gym today as my teeth hurt. I would never have had it done if I'd known.

Saturday, 25 September 2010

Worked out with Emma today. I'll be doing legs on Monday for the last time for 2 weeks because of my varicose veins treatment. Emma had me doing lots of different exercises today, including 180 squats overall.

Yesterday we had a roast dinner and I had 2 glasses of wine. Today I ate some bread and had cheese and crackers, and since I'm admitting stuff on Friday I should also admit that I ate the last 2 kit kats that were in the house. I don't expect to have a good weigh in, and feel quite disappointed in myself, but that's life, that's what it is to be human.

EMMA

But you kept on going...the important thing is you've realised what you've done and you're keeping going so don't beat yourself up too much or you won't move forward again. Take stock, and move forward.

Sunday, 26 September 2010

Today is a new day. I got on the scales and still weigh 12 stone 13, this is still 3lbs higher than 2 weeks ago. That was after 5 days of eating 100% clean, so this is what I have to do. I have 2 weeks until my one year anniversary and I must get to 12 stone 06 so I have hit the target of losing 90lbs in a year, 10 stone overall.

I'M HUMAN

As I read over my own diary entries again I can't believe how I allowed my self to lose focus. I was so close to my goal but with medical treatment I allowed myself to deviate from what I should be eating. I started so well...but we all have a life that interferes in our best laid plans. At least I've remained fairly static, not putting lots of weight on and not giving up.

I will log my food, go to bed earlier and not drink alcohol or eat cheese and crackers. Alcohol and cheese and crackers are my 2 weaknesses. There are now 7 weeks till we go for a day out to Cardiff and this is when I will try on Hudson jeans. I could reach my first target by then, I will reach my target by then!

Today's food:

- **Breakfast**: almonds and a whole juiced cucumber.
- **Mid morning**: protein shake.
- **Lunch**: smoked mackerel and a big plate of salad.
- **Mid afternoon**: half piece of smoked mackerel, 5 cherry tomatoes and some strawberries.
- **Dinner**: whole juiced cucumber, smoked trout and 250g of green beans.
- **Evening**: strawberries.

WEEK 52

Monday, 27 September 2010
Weight: 12 stone 12lbs
86lbs total loss

A very focused day. In the evening I had an apple and water. I was a little hungry when I went to bed at 11pm but resisted temptation and took my zinc and magnesium tabs. I'm delighted to have lost a pound this week, a good poo this morning must have helped! I'm still 2 pounds heavier than 2 weeks ago, though...

It was such a hard day at the gym today - Emma had me doing squats with 8kg weights and this was very hard. I needed to do a good session though because I won't be doing legs for another 2 weeks. My second leg is being treated for varicose veins tonight.

Today I had smoked mackerel for breakfast, turkey and salad for lunch, smoked mackerel and salad for dinner with berries and a Greek yoghurt in the evening. I also ate a portion of nuts so today was a good day, food wise. Early evening I was back at the hospital for my varicose veins op. It really hurts when the needles go in but it should all be worth it in the end!

Tuesday, 28 September 2010

It was hard last night, my legs ached and I felt very hungry this morning. I won't be at the gym today but I will go for a walk later. For breakfast I had eggs and mushrooms, mid morning a small apple and a slice of ham, lunch was chicken with lots of salad!

I'm feeling very tired today, I think it is down to my leg treatment. I ate berries during the afternoon and had salad and steak for dinner, then a Greek yoghurt plus more berries. I was hungry before bed so I just had a very few nuts. I remembered to take my magnesium and zinc tabs this evening.

Wednesday, 29 September 2010

I'm sleeping longer, might be the magnesium and zinc or perhaps a result of my leg treatment. Breakfast was a whole cucumber and a portion of nuts.

I saw Emma at the gym, we needed to make adjustments but it was a good workout, I was feeling tired but still worked with my usual intensity. What I was really pleased with were my sit ups, I did the second and third set without help, I felt very proud of myself!

HEALTHY CHOICES

I was thinking earlier, people often write about being good and then being naughty. One slimming club talks about sins, but I don't think they've got the terminology right. The focus should simply be on making healthy choices rather than making people feel bad about wanting certain tempting foods. Body builders talk about having cheat meals, I think a much better description is a treat meal, where we can treat ourselves to something we don't eat every day, for some people it might be pizza, for me champagne!

So far I've eaten clean on Sunday, Monday, Tuesday and now part way through today (Wednesday).

In addition I've also slept more and relaxed more too. Both of these things are good for me. We went to the cinema and it was just after

11pm when we got home; I felt hungry but didn't eat, I thought it more important to take my magnesium and zinc tablets which need to be taken on an empty stomach.

WATER - IS IT HUNGER OR THIRST?

Sometimes we think we are hungry when we are thirsty. Our bodies cannot differentiate between hunger and hydration which is why we frequently mistake thirst for hunger. It can be worth having a glass of water and waiting 30 minutes to see if the hunger passes.

Thursday, 30 September 2010

I said I wouldn't but I got on the scales today and weighed 12 stone 12 so no change since Monday. Somehow I thought I would have dropped a couple more pounds after being 'good' for a few days. I'm using this terminology even though I know it isn't helpful. I know I ate a bag of nuts yesterday and although they are a good food they are still calorie dense.

I did a joint age assessment I found online. According to my score I am under 30 for all measurements so that's good and perhaps I need to be thankful for what I have.

Lunch today was turkey and salad, dinner was buffalo burgers and salad.

'People often say that motivation doesn't last. Well, neither does bathing - that's why we recommend it daily.'

Zig Ziglar

Friday, 1 October 2010

We had a nice evening meal; steak and green beans. I also had a small glass of wine and a small portion of chips, I know it's not part of the plan, but after enduring the pain of my leg treatment and my teeth I'm feeling pretty sorry for myself.

Saturday, 2 October 2010

Had a lovely cooked breakfast with Simon: scrambled eggs, good quality bacon and tinned tomatoes. Followed this up with smoked mackerel and some tomatoes for lunch. I did get to the gym this afternoon, but it was hard going doing my cardio - I only managed 3 minutes on the stepper and did my brisk walk on the flat, not the incline as normal. However I did manage some of the abdominal exercises - sit ups and

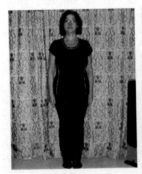 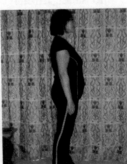 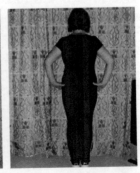

then the pelvic lift crunch where I had to lift my bum off the floor by tilting my hips and crunch my shoulders up at the same time, feel the burn! I did 2 sets of 10 of each exercise and was so very pleased that I did proper sit ups with a slow sit back - Emma was pleased too!

Teeth have been on edge today, not sure why but they have really been hurting and it's driving me up the wall.

More steak for tea, this time just with green beans. In the evening we went in the hot tub. I resisted wine but wanted to treat myself somehow so I had some ice cream, 2 squares of bitter dark chocolate (which might be recommended but are not actually that enjoyable to eat) and then 4 small crackers with cheese. I really think that from now on at weekends I should be able to let up a little, even though I know this won't help me get to my target. It's hard.

Sunday, 3 October 2010

Lovely to have taken my bandage off my leg last night and to sleep last night without my support stocking. I'd planned to go to the gym, but with lunch at Simons parents and having to be at the station by 3.45pm I just won't have the time, not when I want to sort out things in my office as well. I really want to clear the pile of papers on my desk and to tidy out the stack of pending on my front office desk.

MAKING EXCUSES

I can always make time for what's important to me, if I make excuses I'm just disappointing myself.

I had a good lunch, and 2 glasses of wine, then the 4pm train to London to meet Frank for dinner. We ate Thai food and I had ½ bottle of wine, so it was a bit of a carb blitz. I wouldn't have eaten so much at night normally but I always get stressed going to London and then I ate biscuits in the hotel room just because they were there.

WEEK 53

Monday, 4 October 2010
Weight: 13 stone 2lbs
82lbs total loss 4lb gain

I'm in London for a consultancy assignment so the weight readings are from yesterday. I ate a pear and some nuts for breakfast and then had lunch ordered from the Prêt menu. I hadn't realised how little protein is included in a meal. Their tuna salad had only a really small helping of tuna and half an egg, I was really pleased I had some more nuts on me. By mid afternoon I was hungry and ate biscuits and a chocolate brownie. I had to rush for the train so the only food to eat was nuts. When I got home I had a ham sandwich. All in all, a carb rich day. Tomorrow will be different!

BE READY FOR A MISSED MEAL

I always have a 25 gram portion of nuts in my handbag. That means if I am ever delayed or only sandwiches are available I always have something to eat. If I'm away for a day or more I have a 100gms bag in my case, just in case.

Friday, 8 October 2010

This has not been a good week and I've not really been focused at all. Why did I have a big cooked breakfast, then a big Sunday roast, then a meal and 2 large glasses of wine on Sunday? To say nothing of yesterday when I ate a box of savoury crackers in the afternoon as well as steak and chips and more wine. I also haven't been exercising like I used to. I could blame my leg but it is also partly down to the fact that I've remained focused for a year now and I just find it so hard to continue. It's actually been more than a year, such a long time to carry on, it would be so easy to simply say that this is good enough. I'm wearing size 14 clothes, look 'normal', feel fit, yet I still want more. I also fear that I may go back to old ways and within a year find myself being in size 18s again or worse. From today I must log my food. When I used to do this it kept me much more focused.

- **Breakfast**: piece of smoked mackerel and juiced cucumber.
- **Mid morning**: almonds.
- **Lunch**: chicken salad.
- **Mid afternoon**: apple.
- **Dinner**: chicken, roasted vegetables.
- **Evening**: ham and cherry tomatoes.

I went to the *Grand Designs Show* today but luckily I was able to choose a healthy lunch and we did quite a lot of walking about. It wasn't that easy actually to get my lunch, they had lots of sandwiches and only a cheese salad left. I said I had to have salad, told them the story of my massive weight loss and how I didn't want to go off track and they found me a chicken one. This evening I avoided cheese, crackers and alcohol despite Simon having all of these.

Saturday, 9 October 2010

Woke this morning, got on the scales and I'm 13 stone and 1 pound which is 2lbs lighter than yesterday, which has left me feeling better. I will feel better still when I get to 12 and a half stone.

I continue to drink lots of water. Drinking a litre for every 50 pounds of body weight means that at 13 stone I need to drink 3.5 litres, and this is in addition to the water I drink at the gym.

WEEK 54

Monday, 11 October 2010
Weight: 13 stone 2lbs
82lbs total loss, no change

Today I still weigh 13 stone and 2 pounds but on Saturday I had 2 meals out plus I ate 4 biscuits in the hotel and I had a small bottle of cider last night. I've also been eating quite a lot of Greek yoghurt and now I'm wondering if that is conducive to weight loss? Last night I had 3 oat cakes and a few chips. I might have done a fair bit of walking on Saturday but I did nothing yesterday. I really want to beat myself up, why have I eaten too much, I know what I should do and I've failed to follow my own plan! It's not the first time I've slipped back and I really am frustrated with myself.

I saw Emma at 10 and she measured me, I've put on about 0.4cm all over. I think I'm holding fluid so we will measure me again next week.

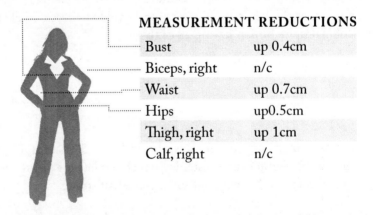

MEASUREMENT REDUCTIONS

Bust	up 0.4cm
Biceps, right	n/c
Waist	up 0.7cm
Hips	up0.5cm
Thigh, right	up 1cm
Calf, right	n/c

Emma and I had a good chat about what I have been eating and I'm going to keep a strict food diary and up the exercise, Emma has advised me to go to the gym twice a day but that's unrealistic with a busy job. Today, all is going well so far:

- **Breakfast**: smoked mackerel and cooked tomatoes.
- **Mid morning**: protein shake after the gym.
- **Lunch**: smoked mackerel and salad.
- **Mid afternoon**: almonds.
- **Dinner**: sea bass and broccoli.
- **Evening**: protein shake.

I worked very hard at the gym today, my legs felt like jelly. In the afternoon I went for a mile long walk.

WHY WE CRAVE CHOCOLATE

We crave chocolate because we lack magnesium. A lack of magnesium shows itself through symptoms which include anxiety, fatigue, headache. The easiest way to get magnesium is through chocolate but we also then get too much sugars and poor fats. Instead we should eat foods such as almonds, avocado, brown rice, cashews, Fish, dark green vegetables, meat, oatmeal, walnuts.

Tuesday, 12 October 2010

I'm keeping a food diary once again to keep track of what I eat. I'm also going to avoid all carbs and fruit for 10 days but don't know what I'll do at the Society of Authors lunch on Friday. I'm also going to make a note in my diary of when I do my exercise each week.

I went to the gym today and did my cardio. Emma gave me a programme to follow consisting of 6 minutes on everything except the stepper which I did for 5 minutes (it is so very hard and I felt like I was about to pass out). On the treadmill I did 3 minutes with an 8% incline and then 3 minutes walking on the flat. I also added in a few exercises, I began with 50 squats and finished with 2 sets of 15 sit ups and reverse crunches, plus another 50 squats. I was really pushing myself, I think most people would think that an hour of cardio was enough, but I have been putting weight on and I feel that shocking my system is the only way to start losing weight again instead of gaining it.

Wednesday, 13 October 2010

I weighed 13 stone and 2 pounds on Monday, yesterday the scales hovered between 13 stone and 13 stone and 1. Today they read 12 stone 12 and I feel much better. I think it's because of 2 things:

- I've been blitzing my body with a lot more exercise.
- I've been very focused on what I eat and drink

My new weight shows you that these things produce results! I've not been hungry. I could easily drink a glass of wine or have had cheese and crackers but doing these things won't get me into size 10 jeans.

At the gym I worked very hard but didn't sweat too much, Emma says that's because my body is used to my programme so it needs to be changed. I worked hard and with one exercise I moved up from using 8kg weights to 10s!

I wasn't able to do the sit ups, Emma said this is because I've over trained the muscles involved. I shouldn't do them each day, it won't reduce the fat around my middle and could lead to catabolism of the muscle.

CATABOLISM OF THE MUSCLE

This means the muscle 'eats' itself to keep going. Catabolism is our enemy. When losing weight, we want to be anabolic, where our muscle are growing and eating calories not themselves!

Thursday, 14 October 2010

I had to see the consultant about my leg this morning. I decided not to go to the gym but to get on with work, but then realised I needed to do exercise so went for a very brisk walk to the shop, over a mile away, and then I walked back carrying all the shopping (an extra 13lbs) in a rucksack.

Friday, 15 October 2010

I had a tasty lunch in the Writers Room at Cheltenham Literature Festival and met some lovely local authors. I was tempted by all the food, puds and drink so I had a couple of profiteroles and 2 small glasses of wine but this meal counts as my carb meal so think this is fine. I wore my faux fur coat and short boots and I looked good.

Tea for tonight consisted of salmon and green beans which are both healthy choices. I then had 2 squares of chocolate which I sucked really slowly. I wouldn't have bought chocolate, but got a free bar from O2.

Sunday, 17 October 2010

I always find it challenging to remain disciplined when I'm outside the home environment.

Today I was on the 15.45 train to London as I have a consultancy assignment. I ate well during breakfast and lunch although steak and salad may have been an excessive choice as I also went out to eat tonight. I also didn't have time to go to the gym or even walk as so much to do before I left. I travel first class and get free drinks and snacks, they put two packs of biscuits in with my coffee and water, and because they were there ... I ate one packet of biscuits, but I was hungry – it had been 4 hours since lunch and I'd forgotten my nuts.

I decided to add some exercise into my day by walking down steps at the tube and up stairs to the second floor in the hotel, and the restaurant was a 15 minute walk away. I told Frank I wasn't going to drink alcohol, then he spotted the champagne cocktails on the menu so I had one. Food was healthy, a good size helping of smoked salmon to start then gilt bream and salad which was tasty. No bread nor pudding.

WEEK 55

Monday, 18 October 2010
Weight: 12 stone 10lbs
87lbs total loss

As I'm away I can't weigh myself today but yesterday I weighed 12 stone 10. I'm now 3lbs short of losing 10 stone since I was my fattest and a 6lb loss this past week. My weight has shot up and down over the past few weeks and I think my dental treatment and leg operation have both impacted upon my ability to stay focused and exercise enough. I'm back to thinking about what could have been ... if I hadn't had these treatments would I be a stone lighter by now?

Since I was again working in London I bought food from the local supermarket to keep me focused. For breakfast I had smoked mackerel and mid morning blackberries. I had some free time so got thinking about goals, I really want to lose 2lbs by the weekend, so I thought about what can I do – eat as healthily as possible, get enough sleep and be very strict about doing enough rigorous exercise; this means both the gym and a brisk walk each day. This week I'm seeing Emma 3 times which will help.

SMOKED MACKEREL AND ROLL MOP HERRINGS

Smoked mackerel is a great food choice as it is an oily fish and contains lots of minerals and great fish oils. It comes pre-packed from the supermarket and has quite a long shelf life so I always keep both this and roll mop herrings in the fridge. Roll mop herrings can have a strong taste because they are pickled in brine. I rinse mine well before I eat them.

I've listed my goals and I'm going to get these up on the wall at home:

	Total loss since October 9th	Total loss since my fattest	Total loss in stone and lbs	MY WEIGHT
Goal 1	90lbs	140lbs	10 stone	12 stone 7lbs
Goal 2	95lbs	145lbs	10 stone 5lbs	12 stone 2lbs
Goal 3	100lbs	150lbs	10 stone 10lbs	11stone 11lbs
Goal 4	104lbs	154lbs	11 stone	11 stone 7lbs
Goal 5	108lbs	158lbs	11 stone 4lbs	11 stone 3lbs

I'm working away and we get treats in the afternoon including millionaire shortbreads and chocolate brownies from M&S. I like these and will usually have 2 or 3 as my treat. I know these aren't good for me however so I must resist but it's hard! It will only be by saying no that I stand a chance of reaching my goals. I didn't get to eat a proper evening meal as I was travelling home, so I had a chicken breast, some tomatoes and some nuts.

Tuesday, 19 October 2010

I was up really early for a radio interview. Later I ate scrambled eggs with tomatoes and saw Simon putting a huge dollop of butter in with them, no! He is meant to use coconut oil. He said that's why his eggs taste so lovely. Late morning I had 2 slices of ham and a couple of tomatoes and for lunch some smoked mackerel and tomatoes, no time for salad.

OILS

Emma told me that olive oil is excellent for salad dressing but when heated it degenerates in quality. Coconut oil on the other hand remains stable when heated so is far better for cooking; and you can use it as a body lotion – double whammy!

I had a good session with Emma today with increased weights and reps. I was remeasured, incredible the difference from last week to this, it really shows how much fluid women hold just before their period. I'm much happier with my measurements today.

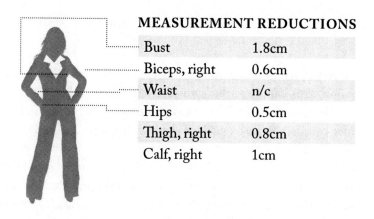

MEASUREMENT REDUCTIONS

Bust	1.8cm
Biceps, right	0.6cm
Waist	n/c
Hips	0.5cm
Thigh, right	0.8cm
Calf, right	1cm

You might think it's odd that I only have the right measurements of my bicep calf and thigh. That's how Ben started with my measurements and I have to compare like with like.

Over the past 12 months my overall drop in measurements are astounding

Bust	From 136.5cm to 102.9cm. Loss of 33.6cm (over 13″)
Biceps, right	From 36cm to 27.6cm. Loss of 8.4cm (well over 3″)
Waist	From 133cm to 93.1cm. Loss of 30cm (nearly 11″)
Hips	From 138.5cm to 107.1cm. Loss of 27.6cm (nearly 11″)
Thigh, right	From 67cm to 53.2cm. Loss of 10.6cm (over 4″)
Calf, right	From 47.5cm to 41.1cm. Loss of 4.9cm (nearly 2″)

Thursday, 20 October 2010

I've stayed focused on eating good, clean food and I had a very good session with Emma at the gym yesterday. Today I bought berries and other healthy food. In the queue behind me at the supermarket was an older couple, she had a pack of Actima yoghurts. I asked if she knew they contained 19 grams of sugar per pot. Like so many people they think if something says it is healthy it is. The chubby lady behind the till said how hard she found it to lose weight and that she'd been to loads of different slimming clubs. I said it was a mental attitude, you have to want to do it. She also spoke about having 4 gin and slim lines a night - low cal soft drinks are as bad for you as sugar.

SUGAR

Highly addictive refined sugar is one of the leading causes of obesity. Many fizzy drinks and health drinks have the equivalent of 5-10 teaspoons of sugar in them. Artificial sugars are worse still. All sugars including honey and fructose create an insulin response and lead to fat storage. A diet drink can make us crave more sweet or carbohydrate rich foods. If we must have something sweet, the best alternative is Stevia, found at health food shops.

Today I bought some size 10 jogging bottoms, they fit! The men's size 34 jeans I have hanging in my wardrobe are far too baggy. I need clothes made to fit ladies now.

WEEK 56

Monday, 25 October 2010
Weight: 12 stone 8lbs
89lbs total loss

Another 2 pound loss. Very hard work out at the gym today with Emma. Yesterday Natalie gave me a pair of her jeans, size 12 from Next - they fit after only a minor struggle with the zip! I am very pleased :)

I've started an Open University course, 'Sports and Exercise Psychology.' We had to introduce ourselves on the course forum, this is what I said:

Why did you decide to take this course? I am very interested in what motivates people to get fit and live healthy. I have made major changes in my life, I have lost 90lb in just over a year and switched from doing the same old thing in the gym to a sustained programme of strength training. I have learnt to love exercise. I want to be able to support others in this area. I'm already a chartered psychologist, (occupational psychology) and see this course as an opportunity to take some of what I already know and use it in a new context, learn new things and possibly offer a new service to my clients.

What's your favourite sport to watch/play? I enjoy working out at the gym and especially love squats and lunges - I impress my friends by being able to do 50 fast squats, or 50 slower ones with weights. I don't watch sport!

What is your favourite biscuit and why? I don't eat biscuits! Full of chemicals and sugar. Possibly an oat cake? (I know I have eaten biscuits every now and again, but I know how bad they are and was making a point!).

Friday, 29 October 2010

Umm, on Wednesday night I had relaxed instead of worked. I had a couple of cheese and biscuits and half bottle of wine. I also had cheese and biscuits last night as well. On the plus side, I did my cardio today. I'm going to be at a conference for the next 2 days, I just realised I haven't put a special request in for food so need to take nuts with me.

Last weekend Natalie gave me a pair of size 12 jeans from Next. Last week they were a bit tight and I had a bit of a struggle to pull up the zip. Tonight the zip went up with no problem and I wore them all evening, not too tight at all. I just need some tops to wear with them, that show off my firm bottom!

Sunday, 31 October 2010

Two days at a conference and it puts me on 'alert' over what I'm going to eat. We had breakfast before we left. I skipped the biscuits at each break but did have a few of the mints in the room over the 2 days. I normally don't like conferences and find talking with new people quite stressful but this time I really enjoyed it. Talking with Simon afterwards we think it was partly because I used to be self conscious over my weight. When you are fat you know that people notice that about you and make lots of value judgements on this. This time I was very confident, it really helps to look good.

FAT PEOPLE ARE JUDGED

Why do people think they can judge fat people and see them as weak and lazy? There are many reasons why people are fat, sometimes it is lack of knowledge. But there are complex psychological factors as well and it is only by addressing these that we can address the weight gain. In the past I compensated on being judged by being really nice and helpful to people. They might be thinking fat woman but at least they didn't see me as selfish.

Lunch was brilliant, a nice buffet so I could have cold meats and salad, and I skipped the roll and pudding. In the evening I had 1 potato and ½ a bottle of wine and chatted with people. Simon had come with me and he told me how good I looked! I am making so much more of an effort, checking out how I look in the mirror, styling my hair, putting on makeup. And I wore my 8cm high heels, I was fine in them all weekend. This sounds a bit shallow but I love the way I look and my figure is now shapely, and all the squats and lunges result in a pert bottom.

Back home we had steak and sprouts for tea and then I wanted more ... so had some oat cakes, a small piece of cheese and some smoked mackerel, plus ½ bottle of wine, I think I had been quite hyper over the weekend and the wine helped me to relax.

Yesterday I didn't do any exercise but this morning we went for a brisk walk, it was at least 2 miles and glad I got my exercise in today.

NOVEMBER AND DECEMBER 2010
Strong But Feeling Down

'I can accept failure, everyone fails at something, but I can't accept not trying.' Michael Jordan

WEEK 57

Monday, 1 November 2010
Weight: 12 stone 9lbs
88lbs total loss, 1lb gain

I began a new programme with Emma today. I had to do sumo squats. I had to go deep enough to touch a low step and if I didn't touch she didn't count it, it really was horrible. I'll be doing them again today but I know I'll be better as my body will be expecting it. It's always like that with a new exercise.

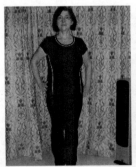
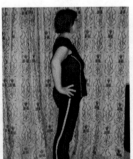
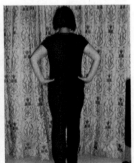

EXERCISE EXHILARATION

I love the feeling I get after exercise. I don't feel worn out but recharged. When I first started exercising I felt knackered but as I got fitter and I could work out even harder I grew to love the feelings of power and strength exercise gave me.

After spending the weekend at a conference my head is still buzzing with ideas. There was so much work to do when I got back. I ended up working on Monday till 1am then I couldn't sleep so I got up and worked till 3 am. I then woke at 7am. I know this isn't good for me and so need to make sure I relax on Tuesday evening. Yesterday morning I did a cardio session on my own, I think I was a bit hyper from work so I really went for it, 6 minutes on each bit of kit and then 2 sets of arm exercises: Tricep dips x 12, straight arm pull down with 17kg x 15 reps, curl and press x 12 with 6kg.

Tuesday, 2 November 2010

Last night my final client left at 6.45pm and I hadn't asked Simon to cook so we went for a curry. It wasn't an ideal food choice but it helped me relax. I had a pint, enjoyed my food and then relaxed more in the evening. I did sleep well last night - 7 hours is a good sleep for me!

Tonight we had soup followed by stew but there wasn't a lot of meat in it so my protein intake was lacking. I think that's what drew me to cheese afterwards, but only 1 cracker - I needed more meat! I had one glass of wine, I wanted it but this isn't helping me to lose weight.

I really hate it when my weight goes up and it keeps happening. I'm beating myself up for it but this is not a good approach. I've got to focus. Seeing the reading on the scales increase makes me feel like a failure; I've been on this crusade for more than a year. I shouldn't be having slip ups and setbacks by now!

THE REASONS FOR FAILURE LIES WITHIN

> Am I being tough on myself by saying that I'm failing? I could make so many excuses, I've had medical treatment, felt low, it's hard because I have less weight to lose, I've done well so far so it's okay to ease up ... I can tell myself whatever I like but ultimately I am the one responsible for my own progress or lack of it.

Thursday, 4 November 2010

There was an article in my local paper titled *'Over 50s get fit and feel healthy the fun way - thanks to new active and able courses'*. The article talked about how learning gentle exercise can help people maintain their mobility and independence, helping them walk upstairs unaided... to make getting in and out of the car a little easier - for those in their 50s? Do people really struggle so much when they are in their 50s? I spoke about this to my young friend Lucy and she said I must feel supersonic, given my level of fitness at my age! I do feel very proud of myself, whatever age we are we should aim to be fit. My dream is that I will still be able to get out of my chair unaided when I am in my 80s. Gosh, I want more than that, I want to still be on trekking holidays well into my 80s and I don't see why I can't still be hill walking in my 90s!

WEEK 58

Monday, 8 November 2010
Weight: 12 stone 11lbs
86lbs total loss, 2lb gain

Just back from a weekend away in Leeds visiting my nephew, Oli. I ate and drank more than normal but this is the start of my husbands' holiday so I think this is fine. Saturday went well to begin with, smoked mackerel for breakfast, salad for lunch but then 2 cocktails before dinner then out for a curry where I also had rice and naan bread – you have to, don't you - plus another cocktail and a large bottle of fizzy water. On the Sunday, a good protein rich breakfast but I did eat ½ a sausage. Lunch was a filet of fish at MacDonald's and then an 'all you can eat buffet' with a long island iced tea. My 20 year old nephew loves this sort of food, but I'd personally prefer much less food, really nicely presented. Red Hot buffet was scrummy, so many options to choose from and I didn't over eat, but I did eat more pudding than usual, lots of little tastes of lots of different things.

That's what I don't like about buffets, yes we can eat as much as we want, but we should focus more on what we need. We don't have to eat massive helpings, unless you are a student like Oli.

TIP: Variety makes us want to try everything, so buffets are dangerous.

Today I'm back on track, no sausage with breakfast, just a roll mop and salad for lunch and chicken and veggies for tea, plus a work out with Emma at the gym. Now I'm feeling a bit tired; I really worked hard and there's no way will I be having any alcohol this week, it's all about focus. My mum is with me at the moment and asked me if I always felt like going to the gym. Always!!! I never have to motivate myself to go, I know I have to go and I also love to go. On reflection it was hard at first because I was embarrassed about my size but as my fitness level quickly increased I loved the way I could challenge my body and see the results as I moved heavier weights.

Tuesday, 9 November 2010

I went early to the gym to get it out of the way - cardio plus 3 sets of 3 arm exercises. I knew I had worked very hard. Most days I want to go but sometimes life is so busy and I could do with spending the time on something else. This is where I practice 'self talk' and remind myself how good I will feel once I have completed it and how each gym session moves me just a little bit closer to my goal. I felt like I had worked very hard. When I got back Simon said that there had been a topic on The Today programme about how women's bottoms are spreading - not mine!

THE POWER OF A SHOWER

Sometimes when I've been busy I've skipped the post work out shower, planning to have it later when I get home. But the strange thing is, when I've had my shower I don't eat as much! I think it 'completes' my workout and the positive ions from the shower make me feel good. It's a great way of looking after myself, including the gentle massage of body lotion I give myself.

Saturday, 13 November 2010

I've put on 3lbs in the past 2 weeks and I've been hovering between 12 stone 08 and 12 stone 11 for a month. I'm annoyed with myself, It's all down to me - I've had too many meal outs, drank too much alcohol, too many puddings. 3 pounds is not a massive amount and I know if I eat carefully over the next couple of days I'll be back at 12 stone 08 but I want to get to 11 stone 11 and I want to be there by Christmas so need to think about what will get me there in 6 weeks.

MY MANIFESTO

- I need to continue with my gym visits plus a very brisk walk every day.
- I need to log all my food and not touch alcohol or cake till Christmas.

- I must avoid cheese and pate, I do love it and I've been eating too much of it.
- I will continue to drink 6 pints of water each day (I never have a problem with this one!)
- I must take zinc and magnesium tabs before bedtime and be in bed by 11pm each night, too often I forget.

Yesterday was a very busy day. I had to leave at 07.30 to go and see the dental technician who will make my crowns, we then went to Cardiff. I can't remember ever shopping like I do now, looking around the stores and seeing what really appeals. I can look at some clothes and think they would really suit me and ignore other clothes that don't match my style. I'm fast becoming the well groomed chic Parisian woman. I'd been interested in buying a watch and had seen a lovely one by Thomas Sabu, I loved it because it was sparkly and a bit quirky but it was £500. In Cardiff I saw a very similar watch by Foli Folie which really was lovely and was around £100. Simon bought it for me as a present. He also bought me a beautiful ring - just costume jewellery but with a lovely sparkly stone.

Sunday, 14 November 2010

At the gym one of the other members told me how great I looked and asked me how I was getting on. I said I had plateaued but that it was my fault because I was eating and drinking that bit more than I should. She told me that one of her friends had lost a lot of weight and had now lots of loose skin but mine was all firming up, she's been watching me over the months and thinks I look so much younger now.

EMMA

I remember training one of my younger ladies on the mat next to Denise who was grunting and huffing with her weights (good lass!), and my client couldn't believe the amount of weight Denise has lost because her arms are toned and smooth not saggy! I explained 'that's the Power of Weights!' She promptly picked up a heavier one, greatly inspired!

WEEK 59

Monday, 15 November 2010
Weight: 12 stone 9lbs
88lb total loss

Really pleased I ate healthily yesterday and I'm on track today. I ate 2 boiled eggs for breakfast, had smoked mackerel and salad for lunch followed by sea bass and salad for tea. I also had 2 mandarins, 2 apples and some raspberries. No alcohol.

I'm so pleased to have lost the 3lb and to be back at 12 stone 09. I HAVE to lose 2lb a week between now and Christmas to meet my target so I'm going back to logging everything I eat. Looking back, I've eaten quite a bit in excess of what I normally eat and I've had quite a few meals out.

I went to the gym and did more of each exercise I did last week, always upwards.

LOSING BELLY FAT

When we put weight on it tends to accumulate on our belly/tummy first. Unfortunately, this will also be the last place it come off!

Wednesday, 17 November 2010

Yesterday I did cardio, today I had a session with Emma. We swapped things round I started with the exercises I normally do at the end when I'm tired. As usual, Emma increased the weights used so I'm now doing lunges with 10kg in each hand and step ups on the bench with 5kg in each hand. I do love my exercise, but I do grunt, Emma makes me work so much harder than I do alone, and I work hard on my own! Another gym member said she was glad that Emma wasn't her personal trainer, as Emma worked me too hard, she was quite shocked when I told me how much weight I had lost.

EMMA

Train hard or go home!

SWEARING

I've often wondered why I swear a lot at the gym when I'm pushing myself hard. Research by Richard Stevens has found that swearing helps us to deal with pain and so grunts and cusses helps us to raise a heavier weight. I've noticed the majority of Emma's clients swear...:)

Today I cooked venison in red wine and then had a small glass followed by 2 x cheese and biscuits - umm not so good but the past couple of days were perfect so this is probably okay and I'll be doing a serious work out tomorrow. Umm, no it's not okay, stop kidding yourself Denise ... I need to stop talking myself into breaking away from my routine.

Friday, 19 November 2010

I have done a lot of exercise this week. What I do is light years away from the 'gentle exercise' or cardio that most people do. You really have to push yourself hard to lose fat. One stumbling block is the fact that most people think that because they have worked out they can have a chocolate bar. What happens is that they put on more calories then they have used up.

I was talking to Jo the other day who is lovely and slim but craves chocolate and wine and only does cardio. She had her body fat measured and she is at 38%. I'm sure that's more than me. The good thing about strength training is it builds up muscle which speeds up your metabolism, meaning you burn through calories even whilst at rest.

Saturday, 20 November 2010

Last night I was working with clients till 19.45 and I knew I wanted a proper relax so I had a couple of glasses of wine, and also duck, not a great idea as it is fatty. I then had 3 crackers with cheese on them. Sometimes you just need to have a relax, but today I will get back on track and I'm off to see Emma again at 10.

Feeling knackered after working out with Emma. My legs felt like jelly once I'd finished thanks to the 40kg deadlifts I was doing.

WEEK 60

Monday, 22 November 2010
Weight: 12 stone 6lbs
91lbs total loss

On the scales this morning and I'm 12 stone 06, I've never been so low and I'm absolutely delighted. I'm also not going to weigh myself till this time next week. I know what usually happens, I jump on the scales, see I've lost 2lbs feel good, have a treat ... weight goes back on. I've now also lost over 10 stone in weight. I want this up in lights, I've lost 10 stone!

As I get smaller I'm so much smaller and take up less space, but I am far more visible.

As a fat person I tried to vanish, I didn't own the space I walked in, I was apologetic for who I was and if I had a cloak of invisibility all the better. As I got slimmer, in particular when my weight dropped below 14 stone, I had so much more confidence. I didn't mind being looked at and knew I looked as good as many. Now that I've crashed through the 10 stone loss barrier there is no stopping me, I own my space, I look good, I'm bursting with confidence. This is a superb feeling.

Thursday, 25 November 2010

I've been far too busy over the past 2 days which I've spent in meetings. I saw someone I hadn't seen for ages, she couldn't believe how heavy I was (for my new size!) and thought I weighed under 10 stone. This is because I'm so muscular. I got delayed coming back from the meeting as the train didn't turn up so I got hungry and ended up having a plain scone. I know it was full of carbs but I needed to eat and it was that or cake. I was quite stressed last night and drank half a bottle of wine.

I did my BMI measurement the other day, I'm no longer obese, my BMI is now 28.6. This is brilliant, I'm now classed as overweight, and I know many sports people fall into this category. I really am so very fit and healthy and I am on top of the world!

Today I went and did a cardio session, the weather was cold and snowy but I needed to do it. I've got stuff going on in my life so I'm feeling quite stressed and anxious, I know this isn't good and it can really impact on my weight loss if I let it. I have to stay calm.

Friday, 26 November 2010

Had a session with Emma and she also weighed me. I'm pleased that I've lost 1.5cm on my hips.

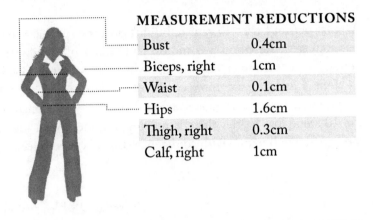

MEASUREMENT REDUCTIONS

Bust	0.4cm
Biceps, right	1cm
Waist	0.1cm
Hips	1.6cm
Thigh, right	0.3cm
Calf, right	1cm

WEEK 61

Monday, 29 November 2010
Weight: 12 stone 5lbs
92lbs total loss

Lost 1 pound. I've been down because of personal stuff and this can easily impact on what we eat. There isn't lots of high fat food in the house so the extent of my 'pig out' has been some oat cakes and cheese. On Saturday I was in a meeting in London. We had to stay in London the night before the meeting and the room came with breakfast. I was almost tempted by croissants but stuck to a yoghurt and 2 boiled

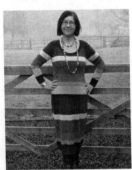

eggs. Alas, I hadn't thought about lunch and I could only get my hands on sandwiches. I just ate 3 small ones (which wasn't ideal) and this led me to eat a couple of biscuits in the afternoon. Lots of people came over to comment on my weight loss and I knew I looked good wearing clothes which show off my trim figure. There was a wine tasting event afterwards but I didn't drink much wine.

No exercise on Saturday or Sunday as we were having photos taken in a family group. Today I did strength training on my own, it really is hard but I know I need to do it. If I'm honest I know that I usually enjoy strength training but I am simply going through a low period right now.

Friday, 3 December 2010

Oh dear, not a good start! I've been unwell and so has Simon and although he has stopped eating, I'm really hungry. I know from the past that there is a connection in our brain that means that when we are in pain we feel the need to eat and this has led me to up my carb intake. Toast and oat cakes. Hardly stuffing my face with cake but still ... I just don't feel satisfied in my head without carbs. Yesterday I asked Simon to get me some boiled sweets (blackcurrant and liquorice) as I thought this would be good for my poorly throat, but I didn't suck one an hour or so and instead went through most of the bag in the afternoon and evening. Overall this week has been hard. I felt too ill to go to the gym but I did manage to go for a short walk yesterday. Better than nothing.

I also have a pain at the top of my bottom and think that when I struggled to lift the weight on Wednesday I might have pulled something.

DO YOU WANT TO BE A SUMO WRESTLER?

I read recently how Sumo wrestlers get fat for their sport. They skip breakfast and eat very little during the day. They eat the bulk of their food in the evening and then go to bed. Unless we want to be Sumo wrestlers we need to eat 6-7 meals each day to help our body burn fat steadily.

WEEK 62

Monday, 6 December 2010
Weight: 12 stone 5lbs
92lbs total loss, no change

We spent the weekend in Oxford. Neither of us were feeling 100% and as it was rainy and incredibly crowded we lazed at the hotel rather than spend our time stomping around the sights on the Saturday. We had cocktails in the Morse Bar before dinner at The Randolph. I started with 2 slices of bread as I was hungry followed by a cheese soufflé. This was not the best choice but I hadn't had one for years and as we were spending a lot of money on this meal I was going to have what I wanted. My main course seemed huge. In reality it wasn't but my appetite is so much smaller these days that it seemed like too much. I left all my potatoes and even some of the meat. We were on a 3 course table d'hôte menu and I chose the chocolate option for pudding, big mistake because it was so rich I could barely manage a spoonful.

On Sunday we had a cooked breakfast but I could only eat half the scrambled egg, I think they make it with cream. We skipped lunch as we were having afternoon tea. We have really enjoyed this in the past but only this time did we realise just how sweet everything is, just a few sandwiches then 2 scones and 4 cakes each. We left quite a bit, I don't think we will be having afternoon tea again.

My exercise consisted of walking around the Ashmolean Museum, better than nothing but with 2 days consultancy coming up I realise that it will have been a week since I was last at the gym.

I got up really early for the train down to London. There was no coffee on the train and I ended up in a freezing cold building. I wish I had my fat to keep me warm! I'm being very sensible with my food this week. Ham for breakfast, chicken and salad for lunch. Plenty of going up and down 3 flights of stairs, both for exercise and to keep my circulation going.

Friday, 10 December 2010

It's always harder to stick to sensible eating when I'm away from home and I've just spent 2 days in London. I try so hard but can be tempted easily, especially by the chocolate brownies they serve as afternoon snacks. I ended up eating 3 over the two days. With that said, I did do as much walking as possible up and down 3 flights of stairs.

On Wednesday I went for my session with Emma and told her about how my coccyx hurts, she said it probably had nothing to do with the exercise I had done but I'm not so sure. To protect my back I did leg presses with 120kg instead of squats but then moved onto cardio. Because I'm not feeling 100% it was hard doing 12 minutes on each piece of equipment and I stopped 5 minutes early. Emma said that many people are getting strains etc. due to the gym being so cold. I went back to the gym on Thursday and I've really worn myself out so I'm having a rest day today, it's really not a good idea to make myself ill by overdoing things.

On Wednesday I was very careful about what I ate - bacon for breakfast, houmous and carrots for lunch, venison and green beans for tea and that was it. Yesterday; egg and bacon for breakfast, houmous again for lunch and duck and carrots for tea. In the evening I had some frozen yoghurt and 3 oat cakes and cheese. I was slightly worried when I got on the scales. I've drifted away from my 6 meals a day and gone back to eating 3 conventional meals a day, maybe I now feel that I should eat like everyone else because I've cracked the 10 stone loss barrier?

TIP: Change plate size from 12 inch to 10 inch. There's a famous experiment where people are given different sized containers of popcorn. Give people a bigger tub and they eat more.

WEEK 63

Monday, 13 December 2010
Weight: 12 stone 3lb
93lbs total loss

Two weeks ago I weighed 12 stone 5, today I'm 12 stone 3. Only 6lbs to go until I've lost a total of 150 pounds, (10 stone 10 pounds)! I really am close and I could be there by the first day of January - it will be such a great feeling.

Another highlight of today was buying a size 12 non stretchy top from Next and finding it fits me fine! Despite all of the good things I've just mentioned, I am feeling quite low at the moment, I have a history of depression. Previously when I'm down I've eaten lots of sweet stuff, this time the worst I did was have three quarters of a tub of frozen yoghurt over a day. This amounts to about 450 calories and it could have been so much worse. In the past it wasn't unusual for me to eat 8 mars bar ice creams or a large slab of chocolate and 2 bags of sweets. I'm a bit achy and a bit tired. Maybe I've been working too hard – actually, there's no maybe about it! Yesterday I didn't go to the gym but I did do a very brisk walk.

Losing so much weight makes it much easier to move quickly. When Simon comes home from work I dash down the stairs to let him in. He now says I move like a gazelle rather than an elephant. I used to thump, thump as I move but now I feel much lighter in my steps, which of course I am. I do love it when I get comments like this and want to save them up and wrap myself in happy feelings. Being low, it's even more important to be reminded how good I look, but people don't know what is going on inside me. I don't share all my feelings with Simon as he thinks I should stop thinking about stuff, but it is hard.

PUBLIC TOILETS

These can be a nightmare when you are very fat. Where it was possible I used to go into the disabled toilet to give me more room. I used to moan to myself about cubicles not being as big as they used to be but I think it was more down to me being so large. I've literally touched the walls with my body as I've sat on the loo and really struggled to get in and out of the door. It was very embarrassing.

15 December 2010

What was going on yesterday? I was so hungry that I ended up eating a full bag of nuts then I had toast after my evening meal. Later I drank 2 glasses of brandy and babycham and a large glass of wine. I didn't do any exercise either but I've been so stressed I needed to be able to unwind and this helped. Today will be a new day, however. Going to the gym with Emma later this morning.

STRESS

I use alcohol and carbs as my drug of choice for dealing with stress, I need to find a better way. I wrote earlier about the importance of staying calm (see Monday 15 March 2010) and this advice is relevant here. I don't always do what I know to be correct however, but I do it more often now than in the past.

Emma: We all have emotional triggers that cause us to eat the wrong things. The secret is to identify these triggers and deal with them.

EMMA

You need to take yourself in hand. What happens is that when you are close to a goal you think this is close enough and so are less hungry (forgive the pun) to succeed. You must focus. When you get close to your goal it is easy to lose focus and talk your self into being happy with your current state. You know you can do better, you can get there.

WEEK 64

Monday, 20 December 2010
Weight: 12 stone 6lbs
91lbs total loss

Bloody hell I weigh 12 stone and 6 pounds today. That's an increase of 3lbs but I have been eating more carbs and drinking alcohol. It is so very cold and the snow means I can't get to the gym which is really not helping. I'm also depressed and trying not to let it show but my body knows how I feel.

Wednesday, 22 December 2010

So much for being strict last night, I had 3 crackers with pate and half a bottle of wine and then half a big bag of crisps. At the gym I did a weights session with Emma. It was hard going because I haven't done much exercise in the past week because the weather has been so bad. I told Emma I'd been eating carbs and had put weight on.

Of late I've been drinking diet bitter lemon, and sometimes two bottles a day. I find it very refreshing, but I had forgotten about the aspartame which makes one crave carbs, so this has not been a good move. So for the next 3 days I must be fully focused, that way I should have undone the damage by Christmas morning. I'm feeling much happier today, I've done lots of good things and no carbs except in fruit. Probably my diet isn't helping my depression.

> **IS THE HARDEST PART GETTING TO THE GYM?**

No, it's remaining fully committed to working out at peak intensity. Showing up and going through the motions is not enough. No one can do it for me, I have to give 100% to my exercise

WEEK 65

Monday, 27 December 2010
Weight:????? Too scared to get on the scales

I haven't written in my diary for a few days and have not made good choices about what I eat and drink. I'm still feeling low and I've turned to carbs. I had so hoped and intended to reach my goal by the end of 2010 but it clearly won't happen. But that's life, things get in the way and I'm human. I need to re-evaluate how I deal with these situations. I haven't pigged out as badly as I have done in the past but I've been eating cheese, and pate, drinking wine and more. Yesterday I bought a gorgeous crusty loaf and ate about half of it. It would be okay if it was my carb day, but at the moment every day is a carb or alcohol day.

Tuesday, 28 December 2010

Today has been a better day. I went to the gym for the first time in 4 days to do a session of cardio. Before Christmas I did a cardio day on the 23rd followed by some strength training on the 24th. I had planned to start writing this book over the Christmas holiday but now with my set backs I'm wondering if I have a story to tell.

EMMA

You do have a story, its real, it's happening; you stumble but you get back up and start again, that's the secret to success. Remember, keep your eye on your goal, never let it out of your sight and you WILL get there.

Maybe it can be helpful to think about how far I've come. Over the past year I have dropped down a size in my shoes because my feet aren't as wide. I can wear my engagement ring again and my three gold bracelets now fit my wrist. I wrote earlier about how fantastic I felt when I could not only buy a womans' watch, but actually had to have links removed because my wrist was so small. It is now much easier to get in and out of cars. When I was fat, I always had to be careful where I parked the car to ensure I could get in and out. If I parked in a normal space with a car next to mine then there wasn't enough space to open the door and get out. I had to change my car to a 4 door model as the doors were smaller!

Thursday, 30 December 2010

Today is a new day, I'm really not sure what happened yesterday. It started well and I did a good work out with Emma but then got focused on work, got the munchies, found malt loaf and ate it! Then there was some chocolate, It's good chocolate with 70% cocoa but I still ate it all, then after our meal I had some Tia Maria to finish off the bottle! I followed this with cheese and pate and crackers. Looking back, it would have been better to put the pate in the bin rather than eat it, but it was lovely duck pate and I did enjoy it.

TIP: A minute on the lips, a life time on the hips.

Today I'm more focused. I've gone back to taking psyllium husk after my food. I haven't been able to get to the gym today because I've been waiting for an engineer to repair our gas fire. Instead, I found a moment to go out for a brisk walk. I've been eating sensibly today: 2 boiled eggs for breakfast; a slice of ham and tomatoes mid morning, chicken and veggies for lunch and finally tea and a slice of ham in the evening. I need to get back to eating like this.

Friday, 31 December 2010

Bloody hell, got on the scales this morning and I'm at 12 stone 10. This is a 4 pound increase and I'm so very disappointed in myself. If I'm being honest, this was to be expected and I didn't weigh myself on Monday because I knew this was going to be the outcome. I'll make sensible choices this evening at the New Years Eve Party. Looking back, I've eaten lots of cheese and biscuits and drank lots of alcohol. I've also done less exercise what with the poor weather and Christmas.

I'm not ending this year on a high but I think this is a realistic account - I really think I failed to meet my end of year target because I got so close to my goal and I thought this was close enough. After feeling so low about personal matters recently I've been drawn to food. On the plus side, I fully expect to have lost 5lbs by this time next week as much of the excess weight I have put on recently will be a result of my body holding water from all the bread. I still have to face up to the fact I ate a lot of chocolate and chocolate contains not just carbs but fat. I ate After Eights on Christmas Day and 3 bowls of trifle plus I finished off the 2 bars of 70% cocoa chocolate. I only needed a little bit for the trifle top but bought 2 bars as they were on offer. The more I think back the more I can think of times I ate more than I should. I had some biscuits with Simon's mum after a difficult email, several half bottles of wine, a few glasses of Tia Maria (to use it up) and a lot of cheese and biscuits.

Anyway, what is done is done. Time to move forward and I now feel very much more focused.

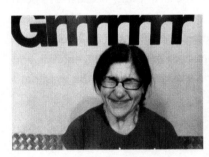 I just got back from my session with Emma, she increased many of the weights and it was hard but I did it. That's why I use a PT to push me so much. It was really hard, as I grunted she said "SHOW ME YOUR WAR FACE".

I am going to be fully focused for the next 2 months and I will log everything. I will go back to basics and stop eating cheese and I will have a carb day every 5 days. I will follow my plan. Tonight, though, I am going out so I will have a glass of champagne but I plan not to eat anything from the buffet.

TIP: Protein keeps you feeling fuller for longer.

Post script: I had a lovely evening at the local pub, casino night. I mainly drank fizzy water, apart from one glass of champagne. I did have a small helping of curry with rice and a few chips. Then a tomato juice. All in all I did very well considering this was New Years Eve. I didn't get silly and drunk and I won first prize, making the most money on the roulette. This was probably because I was the only sober one.

'Success consists of going from failure to failure without loss of enthusiasm.'

Winston Churchill

Saturday, 1 January 2011

I weigh 12 stone and 9 pounds. Time to refocus and get serious. We go on holiday in 10 weeks and I've got lots of clothes to buy. If I shop 3 weeks before I go that gives me 7 weeks to lose 12lbs and to reach my goal of losing a total of 150lbs. I should do it if I follow the key paleo principles, look at the appendix if you need a reminder.

I'm going back to carb cycling. I will only eat carbs after 6pm on each fifth day. When I used to do this I had half a bottle of champagne as my carb meal along with some potato or bread.

Family visit today. As soon as we arrived I was offered a G&T then I was brought a glass of wine. Other people can unintentionally sabotage

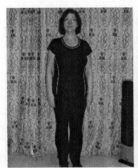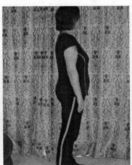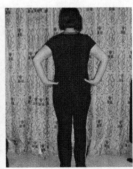

us but I held firm. I was told I could start my diet tomorrow. No I could not, and it's not a diet, it's a healthy eating plan! Today is my first day. I want to get to 11 stone 11.

PEOPLE WILL TRY AND SABOTAGE US

If we tell people we are on a diet some will look for ways to stop us succeeding. It's not always a conscious decision on their part but if they see us getting slimmer and more attractive there may be feelings of jealously and they may think we are showing up **their** failings. It's far better to say we are eating healthily and making healthy food choices.

Today's food:

- **Breakfast**: 2 hard boiled eggs.
- **Mid morning**: slice of ham and 6 cherry tomatoes.
- **Lunch**: steak and vegetables, mineral water, 3 mandarins.
- **Mid afternoon**: 11 cashew nuts.
- **Tea**: 1 roll mop, 9 almonds, salad.
- Lots of water!

It's now nearly 7.30pm and I'm feeling tired as we went to bed late last night. Normally at this time I'd have a glass or two of wine and then cheese and biscuits but I have to break this pattern. It's not easy but I'll feel good on Wednesday when I can have my carb meal.

Sunday, 2 January 2011

I now weigh 12 stone and 8 pounds. I know that you shouldn't weigh yourself each day but just for this first week I will. I am so determined to stay focused and to get to 11-11 asap.

- **Breakfast**: kipper and tomato juice.
- **Lunch**: roll mop and tomato.
- **Post gym**: protein shake.
- **Mid afternoon**: 2 slices ham and apple.
- **Dinner**: roast beef, roasted carrots in coconut oil, cabbage.
- **Evening**: slice of ham, 4 mandarins, 9 almonds.

I did a cardio workout at the gym. Same as usual: 6 minutes on each piece of equipment. I've been doing the same routine for a while now but as I'm now going to be doing this 3 times a week I will need to increase the intensity each week or I feel I may be missing an opportunity.

GET ACTIVE

Find a means of moving and getting more activity into your daily life. At my fattest, I wore a pedometer and went walking, building up the distance I walked over time. It's good to know where you are starting from so take note of what you are doing when you first begin. You may be quite shocked how little it is and you might be inspired to start adding a little more exercise into your day until you build up to 10,000 steps. I'd reached a daily average of 18,000 steps by the time I joined a gym and realised I needed to take things up a level.

I could have easily drunk wine and eaten chocolate or cheese last night. It's not easy to stand firm in the face of temptation. Success comes down to having self control and being concerned for the long term - delayed gratification rather than the short term gratification. A bonus of my long term self control is the fact that I am now able to wear nice clothes. We've got a holiday in less than 10 weeks and I can't wait to wear nice clothes and to enjoy having my photo taken.

The newspapers are full of tips on diet and exercise. In The Times James Duigan, PT to Elle Macpherson, says that at his gym he sees clients in their 40s with muscle aches and pains, some lower back problems and problems with their knees. They lack energy and have increasing cravings for alcohol and sugar. Interestingly I didn't have any of these health problems even at my fattest. He also said that middle aged spread occurs in people who do an excessive amount of aerobic work (5-7 sessions) and not enough weights.

WEEK 66

Monday, 3 January 2011
Weight: 12 stone 7lbs
90lbs total loss

Today I weigh 12 stone 7, the scales did flicker between 6 and 7 but this is still 3 pounds heavier than I was at on my lowest. Emma is going to take measurements, I checked and I weighed 12 stone 5 the last time she measured me so round about the same weight. After avoiding exercise because of the bad weather I wonder what my measuremens will be like now? As you can see below, all my measurements have increased. I've done less exercise and perhaps I'm also holding fluid.

MEASUREMENT REDUCTIONS

Bust	up 1.6cm
Biceps, right	up 0.7cm
Waist	up 1.1cm
Hips	up 1.5cm
Thigh, right	up 0.8cm
Calf, right	up 1cm

My food today is:

- **Breakfast**: fried egg and bacon, cooked in coconut oil.
- **Post gym**: protein shake and small portion of nuts.
- **Lunch**: smoked salmon salad, 3 mandarins.
- **Mid afternoon**: small portion of nuts, apple; houmous and carrot sticks.
- **Dinner**: roast beef, cabbage.
- **Evening**: slice of ham and tomatoes.

Emma certainly pushed me today, getting me ready for our holiday. It really was a shock to my body, doing exercises I've never done before. Throughout the day I kept very focused and ate well.

Tuesday, 4 January 2011

I wondered if I should weigh myself today - I did and I'm 12 stone 5, back to the same weight on my last measurement date. Still can't understand why I'd gain 1cm on my bust etc. yesterday ... I must be holding fluid.

At the hairdressers I chatted to my colourist. She is keen to lose weight but she is doing what most people do, starting off with breakfast cereal, not eating enough protein and drinking lots of low cal drinks. I just want to spread the word and show other people how healthy and effective my food and exercise regime is!

- **Breakfast**: fried egg and bacon, cooked in coconut oil.
- **Post gym**: protein shake and small portion of nuts.
- **Lunch**: houmous and carrot sticks, not enough but I was at the hairdressers.
- **Mid afternoon**: cooked chicken and an apple.
- **Dinner**: game casserole with carrots and onions.
- **Evening**: 2 slices ham, 3 mandarins, houmous and carrots.

I ended up in bed at 11.45pm. It's not good to go to bed so late but I had been working late (doing too much!) so I needed time to relax a bit before attempting to go to sleep.

Wednesday, 5 January 2011

On the scales first thing and I'm 12 stone 3, that means I have lost 7lbs in 6 days, proving progress comes when we are focused and eat and work out correctly. This is the lightest I've ever been.

Another tough day at the gym, but I did better than on Monday, programmes appear easier once you know what you are doing. Emma is going to put the weights up next time. I said it was a struggle but she said if I could still do all 20 reps on set 3 I could go up, she expects me to collapse on the third set! I really had to work hard to do 60 deadlifts with 14kg in each hand.

Earlier I had been to the dentist to have my dental implants fitted. It seems so long ago that I started and now I have 3 more teeth in my mouth!

- **Breakfast**: protein shake taken just before the gym because I had to leave early for the dentist.
- **Post gym**: protein shake.
- **Lunch**: game casserole and 3 mandarins.
- **Mid afternoon**: roll mop herring and salad.
- **Dinner**: venison steaks, chips, sprouts and carrots, chocolate GU pudding. 1 single measure of gin and tonic - it is my carb meal.
- **Evening**: 2 mandarins.
- **Plus lots of water**: I haven't been listing it each time as this is something I consistently do. I have a pint glass on my desk and have 2 pints as soon as I wake up. I drink several more through the day, as I drink them I tally them in my diary.

Today is my 5th day of eating clean so I can have a carb meal. When I was doing carb cycling before I was having half a bottle of champagne and cheese and biscuits on my carb day but cheese isn't a carb. I checked with Emma and she tells me that a piece of cake is better.

Thursday, 6 January 2011

I didn't sleep well last night. It was hard to get to sleep and then I woke at about 4am but dozed till around 6am. I have got a lot of work on and I'm getting a bit stressed over it all, but I also think it may be because I missed my magnesium and zinc tablets last night and also my stomach had more food to deal with.

On the scales this morning and I've put on a pound but that's what I expected and I expect it to have gone tomorrow, plus I hadn't had my early morning poo! I was going to skip the gym today but think I will still go as I will get a much more vigorous workout in the gym than I will if I go for a brisk walk. I know how great I will feel when I've finished my workout and because I work out so vigorously I'll use up about 500 calories (as I do every session)!

- **Breakfast:** scrambled eggs in coconut oil with smoked salmon, not as nice as when Simon usually does this with butter.
- **Mid morning:** mandarin.
- **Lunch:** ham salad.
- **Mid afternoon:** protein shake after gym and 1 slice of ham.
- **Dinner:** venison and carrots.
- **Evening:** mandarin; 2 slices of ham, 3 tomatoes.

I ordered some clothes for our trekking holiday and the size 14 Craghoppers fit me comfortably now, but what about when I lose another stone ... and I do want to lose another stone because I want to be half the woman I was. I'm going to order size 12's.

This is what I posted on Facebook: *I commit to losing 14lbs in 9 weeks. I will do everything possible to achieve my goal. I will go on holiday wearing size 12 trekking clothes and be half the woman I was*.

As you can see from my food details, I couldn't be any more focused if I tried. I went to the gym and did my cardio session, this included 6 minutes spent walking up a 10% incline hill.

Friday, 7 January 2011

I stood on the scales this morning and discovered that I've lost the pound from yesterday, so after losing 7lbs in one week I'm back to 12 stone 03. I don't think I should continue with the daily weigh in any more but it has been good to see how quickly I can lose weight if I really try.

DON'T SKIP MEALS

If you skip meals and get too hungry it triggers the production of the hormone Ghrelin, an amino acid peptide that is produced by the cells lining the stomach and the pancreas and whose main aim is to stimulate hunger and the need to satiate it. If this happens you are more likely to over-eat or crave high calorie food to fill you up and cease production of the hormone.

- **Breakfast**: 2 fried eggs and bacon. I don't think I feel fuller for longer with 2 eggs rather than one, interesting, 3 hours on I could do with eating!
- **Mid morning**: slice of ham and tomatoes.
- **Lunch**: smoked mackerel and salad.
- **Mid afternoon**: protein shake and 20 almonds; 2 mandarins, slice of ham, 1 apple small piece of smoked mackerel. I had a very small lunch and working till 7.30pm so I had 2 mid afternoon meals.

- **Dinner**: duck, carrots and green beans.
- **Evening**: 15 almonds.

Sunday, 9 January 2011

Yesterday was my day off from the gym. I was focused all day with regards to my food intake although I probably ate a few more nuts than usual. Today I tried to persuade Simon to walk up Bredon Hill, he wanted to unwind in a sauna so we went to the gym. I did my cardio session, including 8 minutes at 5.5 kph with a 10% incline on the treadmill. It was hard and I had to really push myself. I want to be able to manage 10 minutes on a 15% incline.

Both yesterday and today I would have loved a glass of wine but I stayed strong, I have to lose this last stone then I can switch to maintenance mode and relax a little bit.

Almost forgot, yesterday I bought a woman's fit zipped jacket, (medium) and it was a nice fit. I also tried on a light weight coat on in M&S which was an absolutely beautiful shade of blue, fitted with a flared skirt. I'm going to buy it next week.

WEEK 67

Monday, 10 January 2011
Weight: 12 stone 4lbs
93lbs total loss

No idea why but I am at 12 stone 04 today. I think this is why you shouldn't weigh yourself so frequently, it is misleading to see your weight fluctuate on a day to day basis. Today is my carb evening meal day. During the day I ate well and worked out with Emma. We then went to the local pub for our evening meal. I had a venison casserole with chips and a medium size glass of wine. The meal could have had more protein and we shared pudding. After this I went home and ate chocolate – why? Maybe it was just because it was there! Now it's bedtime and I am quite annoyed with myself.

Tuesday, 11 January 2011

I had planned to go to the gym but my iPhone went faulty so I had to drive to Bristol and that took up all my gym time. As I had a dental appointment in Cheltenham there was no point in going home so I did a bit of shopping and bought a beautiful cornflower blue coat from M&S as well as a size 12 dress from Wallis. Its got some stretch and will be fine ~~if~~, when I lose more weight. I just hope I can keep going and continue to beat temptation.

I worked long and hard and then finally relaxed. I don't relax much at night and felt I needed a drink so I had half a bottle of wine and 4 oat cakes and cheese. This doesn't amount to a huge amount of over eating but I needed it. I know it won't help me lose a stone and I also missed the gym.

Wednesday, 12 January 2011

I was really busy again today and because of work I didn't have time to eat a big enough evening meal. I had meant to have a second portion of game casserole, but I just didn't feel like it. I ended up eating quite a few nuts last night, a healthy choice but I ate too many. On the plus side I did an awesome workout with Emma.

More clothes arrived from Craghopper, I prefer the ladies fit shirts to the men's medium, a much better fit, but I am so unsure about what size trousers to buy. The 12s are too tight, will I be able to lose the weight to get into them? Simon thinks I should opt for the bigger size. Being able to wear ladies fit clothes represents another milestone, I now have a woman's body rather than being a straight up and down barrel.

Thursday, 13 January 2011

I've been more focused today but I have also been very tired. I decided I need to work rather than go to the gym plus I have to be at my computer all afternoon to answer questions online on the Guardian Career Forum.

What has been going on today? All was fine but then I decided to have a glass of low cal ginger ale which turned into a bottle. I then got hungry, ate a slice of cake, some chicken ... then after tea I was still hungry so I had a glass of wine and I had an oat cake with jam. I ate too much and I'm annoyed with myself, absolutely annoyed.

Am I sabotaging myself? I get so close and then take a step backwards... maybe it is because of wondering about what size clothes to buy, I was trying on the 12s and 14s Craghoppers today, or the stress of all the work I have on - I really have taken on too much - OU course, personal branding course, all my client work, plus the need to get my business ready for a month away.

EMMA

You know exactly what the problem is without me even telling you! You drank diet drinks full of aspartame and you know this triggers food cravings!! Here comes the science bit ... Aspartame contains phenylalanine and aspartic acid which stimulates the release of insulin. As you know, spikes in insulin remove all glucose from the blood stream and store it as fat resulting in low blood sugar and cravings! Phenylalanine also inhibits synthesis of serotonin, a neurotransmitter that signals the body is full so you'll eat more so STAY AWAY FROM THOSE DIET DRINKS!

Friday, 14 January 2011

Today is a new day! I need to skip my carb day on Saturday to make up for yesterday. I had 2 boiled eggs for breakfast which is a good start and I'm drinking plenty of water. Made a decision about the clothes. I'm going to buy what fits me now and not to anticipate that I'll lose lots, better to have things on the roomy side.

Back in October Emma told me to go back to basics with my nutrition and to increase my water intake to 3-4 litres per day (I think I was at this level), to take fish oil and eat 6 meals a day with lots of veggies. Also to go for walks, spending 40-45 minutes a day power walking with ankle and wrist weights and a rucksack full of books. I never did it, need to start.

CLOSE TO GOAL

Close to goal, it is easy to lose focus and talk your self into being happy with where you are. This is when you need to be brutally focused.

Saturday, 15 January 2011

Today we went shopping. I love the fact that I can now buy size 12s and 14s. Emma is right, it is so much harder to stay focused when I already like the way I look. I bought high heeled shoes, a cloche hat, 3 light weight jumpers and the most expensive swimming costume I have ever bought, it cost £139 but it's very flattering and looks brilliant. I was tired so we had lunch out, including pudding, then went shopping where I bought some crusty wholemeal bread - I do so love bread and miss it ... I guess you know what happened next - I had champagne, and then toast - I really think I should be able to ease up at weekends.

> **EMMA**
>
> You cannot ease up when you haven't reached your goal, you're only cheating yourself!

Sunday, 16 January 2011

Getting focused again, had a cooked breakfast with Simon but I'm sure he forgot to use coconut oil, then salad for lunch and a cardio session at the gym, I'll be in London for the next 2 days so I needed to do a good session.

WEEK 68

Tuesday, 18 January 2011

Just back from spending 2 days in London on a consultancy assignment. I've eaten more and exercised less, that's what happens when you don't prepare and take avoidance action. It was good to see people who hadn't seen me for ages, they are amazed by my transformation. Lots of people ask me how I've done it, sometimes I say eat less and exercise more, other times I speak about self motivation. It's about all these things, it's about the need to continually keep going.

Sunday, 23 January 2011

I was not surprised to be at 12 stone 05 on Thursday and I was glad to be back at 12 stone 03 yesterday. After my weigh in I ate crusty bread and cheese, my big weakness, but Simon only buys crusty bread at weekends.

I don't have children at home so I don't have the challenge of convincing children to change eating habits. Simon enjoys foods I don't want to eat and it's because he eats cheese and crackers and loves wine that I'm lead into temptation. If I lived alone I wouldn't have these things in the house. Simon is highly supportive and agrees not to have bread in the house most of the time, only buying a small crusty loaf at weekends. Basically we eat the same food, but he gets potatoes with his meals, and they don't tempt me.

Did a good cardio session yesterday and did more strength training today, it really is hard but I did it! Afterwards I succumbed to temptation and ate biscuits on the train. It's sort of my treat, I really don't like working away from home in London and this is probably the only time I eat biscuits. Yesterday we had coffee out but we skipped the cake. I am predominately in control right now.

Yesterday we went shopping, I like shopping! I bought a stripy mid sleeve length T-shirts and 2 faux leather jackets, really hard to decide which one I prefer so I bought both. I so like to shop now!

So close, and so hard - I'm hovering, I want to be below 12 stone by a week Friday. Not just WANT, I must!!!

TIP: Plan - focus - anticipate!

WEEK 69

Thursday, 21 January 2011

I feel so tired today, I've been working so hard, this is possibly the reason I ate so many biscuits. No! I'm just looking for a reason - they were there, I ate them, it's my fault. I'm annoyed because today I got on the scales and I'm 2 pounds heavier than last week and I ate carefully yesterday. Was it worth it, eating biscuits to put on 3lbs in weight? I chose immediate gratification rather than a long term win. I probably ate eight biscuits on each of the two days which adds up to quite a lot of calories.

Some of the biscuits were chocolate chip and bourbon, it would have been so much better to eat a small portion of proper, real dark chocolate.

I don't want this book to be too repetitive. My story so far demonstrates how with focus you can lose the weight but it also shows how easy it is to give in to temptation and to plateau or even put the weight back on. By the end of September I weighed 12 stone 09 and over these past 8 months I've had many ups and downs, my weight fluctuating by 5-6 pounds.

I've hurt my back which has put a stop to serious exercise at the gym. This month I have been doing light exercise and this has seriously set me back. It's like having a sports injury, I lost my focus big time and turned to carbs and alcohol, then every week or so I got strict for a few days resulting in my weight swinging between 12 stone 03 and 12 stone 06.

INJURY

We all get ill and injured from time to time. When we are focused on an exercise programme it can be frustrating, not being able to do what we want to do. Athletes report feelings of loss, decreased self esteem, frustration and anger. The best way for them, and for us to cope is to understand our injury, to have realistic expectations, to be patient and to comply with our rehabilitation and treatment. We also need to have the belief that we will get better.

WEEK 73

Monday, 28 February 2011

A week before we go on holiday. I was meant to be fully focused on being as fit as possible, but I've let things slip and enjoyed my food and drink too much. Thinking back, I haven't done lots wrong but I have been drinking wine most nights and I've been eating bars of plain 85% chocolate. Yes its good for you but that's when you eat a couple of squares, not a whole bar. What got me started on the chocolate was finding out that Green & Black's Maya Gold chocolate comes from cocoa producers in Punta Gorda, Belize. That's where my grandmother is from and we will be visiting there shortly but this really isn't justification to start eating chocolate. I usually eat 1 or 2 oat cakes, but I've been eating fruit ones and ginger ones and eating lots more than one or two, I think my record was eight last Monday. This is not good! I plan to eat carefully today but we are going out for a curry tonight.

I'm feeling quite fat around my middle, wondering why ... is it because I'm holding fluid there? Is it because I'm not able to exercise like I normally do because of my back problems? Or, is it down to my increase in food consumption. I know the answer.

WEEK 74

Monday, 7 March 2011
Weight: 12 stone 4lbs
93lb total loss

Went to bed at 11 last night and it was after 6 when I woke so all in all a better nights sleep. Got on the scales this morning and I'm 12 stone 4 so I'm pleased. It would be great if I can lose another couple of pounds before Friday when we go away for a 4 week holiday in Belize and Guatemala.

APRIL 2011

WEEK 79

Monday, 11 April 2011
Weight: 13 stone
84lbs total loss, 10lb gain! (7th April)

We got back home at 12.30pm on the sixth of April. We had a brilliant holiday but I know I have put weight on. I decided to wait till the next day to weigh myself, so I got on the scales first thing and I was mortified to discover that I weighed 13 stone. This means I put 10 pounds on whilst away. Bloody hell! I do know, however, that my body needs to reacclimatise and that a lot of this weight will be water/ glycogen. I felt tired so I didn't do anything, my focus was on getting my sleep right as there's a 7 hour time difference. Better news on Friday. I weighed 12 stone 11. Did my first work out with Emma in 6 weeks and everything was so hard. The 6 weeks of no exercise came about because there were 2 weeks where I couldn't work out as extensively because of my back problems and then we had our 4 week holiday.

Despite having an active trekking holiday I still came back 10 pounds heavier. There was a lot of stodge in the meals, I ate less veggies and I also ate cake, ice cream and alcohol. Plus, even though we were trekking through the jungle in Belize and walking up Mayan temples, the physical activity wasn't as sustained or as challenging as my workouts in the gym.

Saturday morning I woke and could barely walk. With squats and lunges my body was doing things it hadn't done for ages and this meant it was hard even to sit on the loo. No exercise today because of this. I usually portion control my bag of almonds but today I had the 100gms bag on my desk and got through the lot in a day, yes they are good for us but not in that quantity! On Sunday everything still ached, I had planned to go to the gym but the weather was so nice that I did a brisk walk to the shops and carried 22lbs of shopping back in a rucksack. This afternoon I drank some beer and wine and ate cheese and biscuits. Oh dear.

Today I saw both my chiropractor and Emma and I promised Emma I'd write down everything I ate. I started doing this but then I ate some things I probably shouldn't have so stopped writing.

Tuesday, 12 April 2011

Another bad day today, went to the supermarket and bought a bottle of Gin as well as some chocolate and crusty bread for Simon. For lunch I ate a cheese and pickle crusty roll, then ate the chocolate. In the evening I did a brisk 3 mile walk which is good but I also bought a magnum and had a couple of gin and tonics and some cheese and oat cakes that evening. None of this is productive.

Wednesday, 13 April 2011

For breakfast I had scrambled eggs and bacon. I was off to a good start, then I had a client followed by a session with Emma at 11.00.

It's hard getting refocused after a holiday. I'm still in holiday mode so it's hard to stop drinking and to go back to strict eating. I managed for a couple of days, but for the past day or so I've been drinking G&Ts, eating cheese and biscuits and yesterday I even had crusty bread, chocolate and ice cream. I'm never going to reach my goal if I carry on like this.

Emma gave me a strong talking to today. I've got to put a photo of a fat me on the fridge, as my phone screen saver and on my computer. I've got to go back to the beginning and log my food, but more importantly, that I need to plan what I'm going to eat and plan when I'm going to exercise. I used to do this, and then as I've gotten close to my goal – I was only 6 pounds away from losing the 10 stone 10 pounds (150 pounds) - I began to let things slide. I plateaued and then put weight on while on holiday.

EMMA

You have climbed up the large mountain, and are in sight of the summit. You are thinking that you've done enough, but you haven't yet! You will put weight back on. It is much easier to put weight on than it is to lose it. You've got to get focused again, quickly.

Following my workout I had a protein shake. Lunch was turkey and salad and an orange. Mid afternoon - portion of nuts, 6pm - banana and orange, dinner - pork, broccoli and cauliflower plus a small roast potato and gravy. We didn't eat till 8pm as I put the meat in the wrong oven. I had a can of diet ginger ale in the evening.

Thursday, 14 April 2011

On the scales this morning and I'm 12 stone 10. I had intended to go to the gym before seeing the chiropractor but I just won't be able to go so early and I will be too rushed to go afterwards. I will simply make sure I go on both days during the weekend.

I had a roll mop herring for breakfast, smoked mackerel and salad for lunch then a 3 hour session with a client. After this I got a couple of complex, stress inducing emails and remembered I had a bar of chocolate hidden away in a drawer. I only intended to eat a couple of squares but within 30 minutes I had eaten the entire 100g bar. Why?

Because it was there! I used to be able to resist so why couldn't I resist it today? Late afternoon I went to the shop to collect a package, bought a crusty roll for Simon and again ate it - I loved it, it was so lovely to eat ... didn't have much for tea, just a bit of pork and tomatoes, then I went to the cinema where I ate some frozen yoghurt. This has not been a good start.

Saturday, 16 April 2011

Umm, I think I have fallen into the same trap that many people fall into – I log my food when doing well and conveniently forget to log anything when I know I've done less well. Yesterday, the only exercise I did was in the form of a brief, brisk walk to the shops/cinema. I ate well for breakfast - eggs and bacon, salmon and salad for lunch but going to the cinema I needed to eat. Whilst shopping I bought a crusty roll and ham and as they had half price sandwiches we bought those too and I ate the sandwich at the cinema as I was hungry. When I came back home mid evening the crusty roll called to me ... I resisted the alcohol and had a portion of nuts.

Sunday, 17 April 2011

Today I'm focused. I got to the gym for 8.00 and did a 45 minute cardio session, then went home for eggs and bacon and I'll be having salad for lunch and chicken and veggies for tea.

My workout was very strenuous and I've ate well, resisting wine, beer, potatoes, gravy. It's approaching 9.30pm and I'm going to go into the hot tub, then I'll take my zinc and magnesium tablets and have a good nights sleep.

I just realised I haven't been logging my water. At 13 stone I should be drinking just over 3.5 litres in addition to the water I drink at the gym.

WEEK 80

Monday, 18 April 2011
Weight: 12 stone 8lbs
89lbs total loss

A second perfect day, started off the day by getting on the scales and I weighed 12 stone 8lbs, Emma may be annoyed that I haven't been fully focused but I've still lost 6lbs of the 10lbs I had put on when I was on holiday. I had a roll mop herring for breakfast, not everyone's idea of an ideal breakfast but I can't eat egg and bacon every day, that's a sure ticket for developing an allergy to those foods. I went to the chiropractor and as my knee still twinges a bit he is making an appointment for me to see a physiotherapist. After that I saw Emma. Rob, my chiropractor had told her I could do squats and lunges but once again she had to change my programme on the hoof as it twinged when I did these. Straight leg deadlifts were okay and I was glad to do some leg exercises.

IS SHOWING UP ENOUGH

No, it's remaining fully committed to working out at peak intensity. Showing up and going through the motions is not enough. No one can do it for me, I have to give 100% to my exercise

As usual I had my protein shake after my exercise. For lunch I had a chicken salad, mid afternoon I had ham and tomatoes and finally I ate fish and veggies for tea. We had Simon's friends round this evening and I had to make the sandwiches: cheese and onion in crusty bread - my favourite - but I resisted and had chicken and tomatoes instead. I did drink some diet ginger ale and I know that diet drinks aren't good for me, but they are okay once in a while, I kid myself, and I think late in the day is the best time to have them, if I must, as they can make you want to crave carbs.

Spoke with Emma earlier and she told me I have to stay focused and avoid distractions. Once I hit 12 stone 3 again this is not an excuse to stop trying and I have to stay disciplined until I reach my final goal.

Tuesday, 19 April 2011

Woke this morning, weighed myself again and I'm 12 stone 7lbs today. I've lost a pound but this could be a minor fluctuation, I shouldn't weigh myself every day.

I watched Supersize/Superskinny. The bigger lady is 5'4 and weighs just over 18 stone. She looks huge but I weighed 4 stone more than that at my biggest. When I was very fat, I was also solid so my size doesn't quite match up with how much I weighed, but never the less when I look back at the early photos I realise I was enormous. I'm looking good now and I think that's why I'm struggling to lose the last 10 pounds.

Tonight I had a client session and didn't finish till 9pm. Usually I'd have knocked back half a bottle of wine to relax. Not tonight, just a portion of nuts.

Wednesday, 20 April 2011

Can you have a worse day than I had? My car broke down a couple of miles from where I live and just 40 minutes before I had to collect a client from the station. I'm not an employee who can call the office and get someone else to see a client, I had to get sorted right away. After an initial panic I got the car moved to the pub car park, did a very brisk walk home, organised a taxi, arranged to meet the RAC late afternoon ... I got everything sorted but it was oh so stressful. I had missed lunch (I just ate a few nuts) and although I held out until 9.30pm I then succumbed to a G&T and a glass of wine. It got worse - I also had 2 oat cakes with cheese and then some toast and marmite.

Earlier I had a gym session with Emma. I told her I had a pain in my back, she suggested I take Ibuprofen and also that perhaps I was going too fast on my uphill walking. Instead of going at 5.7kph at a 6.5% incline it would be better to slow it down and take broader strides, that will mean that I don't lean forward, thus not straining my back.

Thursday, 21 April 2011

No car this morning meant I was unable to go to the gym. The car was ready for collection this afternoon so I did a brisk walk to the garage, it took me about 40 minutes. I then went shopping and bought a packet of luxury biscuits. It wasn't huge but I started eating them in the car and had probably eaten half the pack by the time I got home. I then finished them off myself, I didn't want Simon to see a half eaten packet. I had a glass of wine but that was it. Evening meal was sea bass and salad, lunch had just been nuts as I didn't have any salad stuff in the house.

HIDING THE EVIDENCE

Is it a case of 'out of sight, out of mind'? If I hide the wrappers it doesn't count? I know if Simon had seen I had eaten half a packet he would have asked me why I ate so many. On reflection, it would have been better to admit eating half the packet than to make things worse by eating the rest.

Friday, 22 April 2011

It was Good Friday today and we walked up Bredon Hill instead of going to the gym. Breakfast was 2 fried eggs, tinned tomatoes and 1 sausage. Lunch was ham salad, dinner was steak and salad. But then

I had half a bottle of wine and started eating Simon's shop bought ginger cake, which I don't even like. I did eat strawberries which was good but this was not enough to counteract the cake.

Saturday, 23 April 2011

Roll mop for breakfast, a cardio session at the gym, chicken salad and strawberries for lunch and one chunk of crusty bread and butter. I had a glass of wine late afternoon. It's the weekend, Simon's drinking, why can't I?

YOU CAN'T HAVE EVERYTHING

If you want to achieve your goal you can't have it - what do you want?

Sunday, 24 April 2011

Lunch out with family, my food and drink intake was perfect. It really is hard to have a life when you have to be oh so careful, and as I keep on saying, I think I look fine at the moment because I can comfortably fit in a size 14 and sometimes a 12. Do I want to be scrawny? I read in the Sunday Times that women who are a size 14 are happier than those of any other size.

WEEK 81

Thursday, 28 April 2011

I've now been eating clean for 4 days, remaining as disciplined as I was when I first began this healthy living mission. Tuesday and Wednesday have been perfect eating days where I basically just ate protein and veggies. I've included nuts as they help me feel sated. I divide my pack into 4 and had 1 portion on Tuesday and just over a portion yesterday. I've also had sessions at the gym with Emma so I've done a decent amount of exercise.

So far I'm not missing alcohol, maybe drinking it becomes routine so I'm glad that I'm breaking the habit, it's just full of empty calories and it reduces our willpower. I spoke with Emma about my carb meal - crusty bread or half a bottle of champagne - she said I could have 1 crusty roll and 1 glass of wine, maybe that will work? I am looking forward to having this. After today I'll be having a carb meal every 5 days, I used to be satisfied with this and now wish I'd never deviated from this plan.

'You can have excuses, or you can have results. You can't have both.'

Unknown

WEEK 83

Monday, 9 May, 2011
Weight: 12 stone 10lb
87lbs total loss

Today is the first day of the rest of my life. I've had some false starts, been tempted to join the dark side by chocolate and wine and I've tried to get back on track and then got sidetracked again. Every time I've been setback, however, I've picked myself up and started again. I think this is how most people fail, they don't pick themselves up and

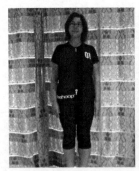 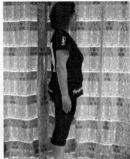 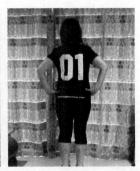

start again, they slip and give up, thinking that as they've had one bar of chocolate they might as well have two. Instead of slipping up and getting back on track they view one setback as a complete failure.

I had an exam last week and I knew with revision comes carb cravings. I gave in to them. On Wednesday last week I started again, had a really good Wednesday, Thursday and Friday but on Saturday I was so very tired, my motivation was lower than it should have been and I picked up not one but two 100g bars of chocolate and then had wine. On Sunday I had yet more chocolate.

SETBACKS

Few people are perfect all the time, so far you've read about the setbacks I've experienced due to medical treatment, setbacks due to sports injuries and set backs due to giving in to temptation and thinking I'd lost enough weight. I have only failed if I don't learn from these events. Setbacks are part of any learning curve. We have to keep going. I've "restarted" my mission every time I've had a setback and when the time is right I will eventually have succeeded as a result of continually getting up and carrying on after a fall.

I'd arranged to be measured by Emma today, I hoped she would forget but she didn't, at least I got to know what the damage was. I now measure more than I did last November. It could be a lot worse but I could also have reached my goal by now if I'd stayed focused. I'm particularly disappointed in the increase around my waist and hips.

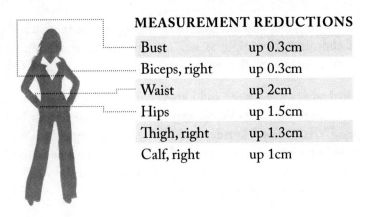

MEASUREMENT REDUCTIONS	
Bust	up 0.3cm
Biceps, right	up 0.3cm
Waist	up 2cm
Hips	up 1.5cm
Thigh, right	up 1.3cm
Calf, right	up 1cm

My best measurements were on November 26, but I lost my focus, sunk into depression and had sports injuries. Overall the increases above aren't huge but it's not good to see measurements going the wrong way. I feel like a failure but I know it was right to get measured so I could assess the damage.

Wednesday, 11 May 2011

Last night I went to a meeting and there were 2 larger ladies. One was eating a big plate of cheese and drinking large glasses of diet coke. She said she was on a diet but clearly was not following good eating habits. I really want to start helping others lose weight.

Today went well, I ate healthily, did a session at the gym with Emma and also walked/jogged to the shops and back. I've started chewing gum, is this okay? It stops me from craving sweet stuff.

I am eating really well, plus I'm now also eating a small punnet of blueberries a day - they are a super food and again help satisfy my sweet tooth. I used to put them in the freezer and think I will do that again. They take longer to eat when they are frozen and I like them this way.

Friday, 13 May 2011

Another perfect day - yesterday I did strength training and today cardio. Today I changed my cardio to 10 minutes on the cross trainer, bike, cardio wave machine, stepper and rower. I also walked at a 7.5% incline. Very sweaty. Feeling a little stressed about my never ending work load so I had a chill out in the sauna.

I'm now leaving to spend a weekend at a festival. We are staying in a hotel rather than camping so this should mean I'm more in control of my food. I can have chicken or ham and tomatoes for my lunch and tea each day. I can't wait to weigh myself on Monday, after 7 days of eating so well. I was 12 stone 11 last Friday, and then had a weekend of carbs and chocolate and alcohol so I must have been at least a pound heavier by Monday. I'm wondering if I can shave 7lbs off. It would be brilliant to be at 12 stone 5, so got to stay focused if I want this to happen.

WEEK 84

Monday, 16 May 2011
Weight: 12 stone 7lbs
90lbs total loss

I had a good time at Bearded Theory Festival, lots of dancing and I was careful about food although maybe I ate slightly more nuts than I should. At a festival you spend a lot of time standing up. My husband found his back was hurting. Not me - I've got a strong inner core!

INNER CORE

The inner core muscle can't be seen, yet they are some of the most important muscles in the body. These are responsible for strength, balance and power. Most importantly, they help with balance and also serve to support our spine and body. With a strong inner core we reduce the likelihood of injury and lower back pain and we have improved posture.

Today I had planned to go to the gym but got delayed with client work. Instead, I went for a very brisk walk to the local shop and carried back 17lbs of shopping in a backpack which I think is as good as a work out. I walked back very briskly as well.

Sunday, 22 May 2011

Today I had my carb meal. I had steak and chips plus two thirds of a bottle of champagne. It then set me off and I had 2 slices of toast and honey as there was nothing sweet in the house. Yesterday I bought some size 12 Capri trousers for the gym, they do look good.

WEEK 85

Monday, 23 May 2011
Weight: 12 stone 5lbs
91lbs total loss

Today I had egg and bacon then went off to the gym. Emma had told me to work through the strength programme on my own. I did and did it well, perhaps I rested slightly more than I would otherwise have but I was manic on the cross trainer, went at a really fast pace as I was listening to banging classic creamfield tunes.

I had planned to go for a walk as well this afternoon, but it was all a bit much because of work. What I did manage though was to walk around the garden about 6 times while I was on the phone to my mum.

Over the past week I've been eating well but still things have crept in. Twice I made casserole with wine - beef with shallots, mushrooms and red wine, and later chicken with white wine.

When you cook with alcohol it burns off so it doesn't count, or is that untrue? In truth, I did have a swig or two while I cooked and the first time we shared the rest of the bottle and the second time I finished it off myself and then had 3 crackers with cheese as it was my carb meal.

On Sunday we visited family, I had 2 glasses of wine at my sisters alongside stuffing and a roast potato with my dinner. Dessert consisted of a weightwatchers lemon meringue pie. Even though it was horrible, I still ate it. Later we went to my mums and I had another 2 glasses of wine but these were small glasses, then with my salad I had some crisps and a bread roll and an M&S pudding. It was from a meal deal but it was horrible so why did I carry on eating it? Both puddings were synthetic in taste, I should eat real food.

Monday I ate well to compensate and on Tuesday I ate okay. I had lunch with a client at the pub with extra veggies instead of potato. For tea I had pork chop and carrots, some blueberries in the evening and then nothing more, went to bed a little hungry, but I was still trying to compensate for Sunday.

Overall this month I've done well with my exercise, I'm going to the gym about 6 times a week now. This is the maximum amount I will go. I could sometimes swap a gym visit for a brisk walk or a slow jog. I have a goal and this intense workout regime is helping me to get there, previously I was only going 4 or 5 times a week. I do need one day of rest a week, though.

WEEK 86

Wednesday 1 June 2011
Weight: 12 stone 5lbs
91lbs total loss, no change

For breakfast I had egg, bacon and tinned tomatoes. Then to the gym where I did 10 minutes on the cross trainer as a warm up before I began my session with Emma. I told her that today I weigh 12 stone and 5lbs and that I have 15lbs to go to be half the woman I was. She wants me to get below 12 stone. I said that if I went off to boot camp I would certainly achieve this as I'd be doing so much exercise. This comment got me thinking as to how exactly I could set up a boot camp of sorts at home:

Emma has suggested:

- Wake up, drink coffee on an empty tum (to help burn fat).
- 60 minutes walk up hill on the treadmill - 8% incline at 5.5kph.
- Breakfast.
- Weights session later on in the day. A brisk walk each evening.

The hour I spend on the treadmill will use up 500 calories a day, that amounts to a pound a week.

At the end of my session I didn't feel knackered so I got on the treadmill, I was really sweating a lot, I managed 50 minutes before I did my cool down, not bad at all!

Lunch - 60gms houmous and carrot batons, 14 almonds; having had 2 coffees this afternoon I moved onto green tea. Dinner - pork with green beans and strawberries.

Thursday, 2 June 2011

I've just got back from the gym. I did my 1 hour of walking uphill fuelled by nothing more than a cup of black coffee. I arrived there just after 6.30am. Today I dropped the incline to 6% as I could barely manage it yesterday and had to hold onto the machine for part of the time. I've set up my Fat2Fantastic Facebook page as I think this will be motivational.

EMMA

You're doing fantastically well chick! keep it up and see you tomorrow! xxx

Last night I ate a small pot of houmous (30g) with lots of carrot sticks and a few cherry tomatoes. I also went for a 20 minute walk so in total I did 3 hours of exercise! All this month I am acting like I'm at bootcamp, but it does take up a lot of my day, so I've got to be disciplined. I have to remember this is all worth it. On Facebook Jo said *'I want your willpower!!!'*

Lunch consisted of a big plate of salad and ham. When I'm busy I tend to graze, I know it is much better to take the time and sit and eat, which is what I'm doing now. I had a massive amount of veggies, now I feel stuffed!

EMMA

On Facebook: I'm so so proud of you for all you've done and all you are going to achieve. I have no doubt in my mind that you will reach your goal. You are an inspiration not only to those battling their weight issues but to me too. Keep going chick I'm right behind you ready to kick your ever decreasing butt around that gym! Love ya x

EAT PROPER FOOD

I don't eat diet foods or drink diet drinks and I don't count calories otherwise I'd be eating a mars bar instead of a piece of mackerel. Same calories, but a very different impact health wise.

Friday, 2 June 2011

This morning I got up at 6.15am, drank a mug of black coffee then spent 1 hour walking at an 8% incline, I have never sweated so much! Afterwards I took the car to the garage and walked home which took 40 minutes. For breakfast I had smoked mackerel and tomatoes.

I'm feeling good although legs ache a bit! Now I'm back home and I'm eating raw green beans - they're tasty and stop me nibbling on other things while cooking.

On Facebook Mark says: 'If you approach this with the vigour you demonstrate in your business life you're onto a winner. Go for it Denise. You've certainly changed since I first saw you back in 2006.'

Friday, 3 June 2011

I woke to my alarm at 6.10am. I had everything I would need to go to the gym ready including a thermo mug so I could finish my coffee in the car on the way. I did just over an hour on the treadmill. Today I changed the incline to 6%, yesterday I'd had to hang on for some of the time and I don't think that's great so I dropped the incline and now I'll do 2 days at 6%, then 2 days at 6.5% etc. I apparently burned off 435 calories (never too sure how accurate this is) so I kept going for another minute to bring this figure up to 450.

I got home and had 2 more cups of coffee. I then had egg and bacon and mushrooms, all cooked in coconut oil rather than olive oil.

LOW FAT IS NOT THE BEST CHOICE

People get very hung up on eating low fat, but low fat usually means high sugar and sugar is far worse for you. Also, people will eat/drink diet products but the artificial sweetener in them encourages you to eat more sugar. If you have to drink cola, it's better to have 1 can of non diet than 3 of diet cola.

I got very sweaty at the gym and my head got very sweaty so I'm going to have to wash my hair each day. I can't use my straighteners each day – well, I could, but it's not good for my hair. What I've done is use big Velcro rollers which have smoothed my hair quite a bit, this isn't the way I prefer it but it's better for my hair. I want to go to the gym again and go for a walk but I'll need to think about how I can fit everything into my day, especially as I'm going out tonight. I think I'll do a 30 minute walk at 12, as I have a client here at 1pm. I'll go to the gym once she leaves and do a 30 minute walk tonight before we go out. This makes for an hour of walking over the whole day.

I went for a walk to the bottom of the village, up to the post box and back home, I always thought this was a 15 or 20 minutes walk. Maybe it used to be but I did it in 12 minutes, I doubt such a short walk made much of an impact of my goal of walking for an hour today.

For lunch I had an enormous plate of salad with smoked mackerel, I even took a photo on my phone.

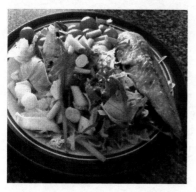

Food like this takes much longer to eat but will fill me up. I've decided that after I do my strength session today I'll do an extra 20 minutes on the treadmill, then I'll just have 30 minutes or so of walking left to do today.

This afternoon I went to the gym again. I did most of my strength training but skipped the squats and lunges, I'm getting a bit worried about my session with Emma tomorrow. My knee just hurt for a moment, so I did well considering, but now I feel so very tired! I wasn't up for a further 20 minutes of walking and as I had work to do I'll not manage 3 hours of exercise today. Am I disappointed - no, because I've still done over 2 hours and I do have work to do as well.

> We aim above the mark to hit the mark.

Today I had my carb meal: we had beef casserole and green beans and then at the cinema frozen yoghurt. I thought about having a glass of wine as well but that will lead me into more temptation.

Saturday, 4 June 2011

Back from the gym. I did an hour of mainly weights with Emma. I then did 30 minutes on the treadmill. 8% incline but dropped the speed to 5kph. I looked a sight by the time I'd finished but after my shower and another cup of coffee, plus a portion of almonds, I feel great. In the afternoon I had a cup of coffee then went out for a brisk walk, a circuit of my local area is 3.7 miles. I took 1 hour, I want to speed up a bit more next time. I have only started drinking coffee temporarily - I need to see if the gain I get by an increase to my metabolism compensates for the increase in cortisol that caffeine causes in my body.

Sunday, 5 June 2011

I went on a very long brisk walk this morning, (4.5 miles) ate egg and bacon for breakfast and ham salad for lunch. I was going to a lunch time party and assumed there would be lots of carbs, which there was, so best to play safe and eat beforehand, It meant I could say no to fattening foods.

On the way home I had a portion of nuts and some blueberries. I was going to do a second walk but it was raining so I wimped out. This did give me time to do some work instead and read the paper. For dinner I had steak and salad and then some more blueberries in the evening.

WEEK 87

Monday, 6 June 2011
Weight: 12 stone 3lbs
93lbs total loss

I'm back to 12 stone and 3 pounds and I'm so pleased. This is the lowest I've ever been and it is good to be back at the cutting edge.

Just got an email: *'I am sooooooo proud of you Denise, I'm sure you are an inspiration to everyone who carries that little bit extra. I wish I had the will power you have.'*

But it is not just about will power, it is about taking sustained action and not letting set backs and eating too much at times take you away from achieving your long term goal.

First thing I had a cup of coffee then spent 50 minutes walking uphill on a treadmill. Next I took 2 hours to shop/work before a session with Emma - mainly weights. Lunch was salad with chicken and houmous. I really like houmous and carrot sticks.

DRINKING COFFEE

I'm currently drinking about 7-8 cups of coffee a day. It's meant to boost fat loss, and it's something I started doing a few months ago, BUT it also stresses our bodies. Today I'm going to cut back on my coffee. I'm going to move to 4 cups and then gradually reduce this to 2 cups over the next few days.

Thursday, 9 June 2011

I am getting tired, possibly because I'm doing too much exercise, twice a day is not sustainable. Today I got stressed over getting my new iPad to work and I've spent a lot of time out at the Cheltenham Science Festival so this evening I'm having a couple of glasses of fizzy wine. Sometimes, rather than planning a 'cheat' day, it's good to just be spontaneous ... actually, who am I trying to kid! One of the sessions I went to was on addiction and many of us change from one addiction to another, so maybe I've changed my addiction from food to exercise.

WEEK 89

Wednesday, 22 June 2011

I read an article in an online newspaper site about a celebrity who has lost 7 stone through a gastric bypass op. There are 73 comments all slagging her off - she hasn't lost the weight, it's the surgeon and they want to read stories by real people who have lost it through their own hard work. I'm so glad I've kept this diary and I hope it motivates you!

This morning I got on the scales and I've put on a pound but our bodies hold different amounts of water from day to day so I'm okay with that. It was good to see a reduction in measurements on Monday.

I was tired today, it's hard doing early morning walking on the treadmill and immediately following this with a weights session. I saw Emma at 11, not sure why but today my knees hurt so we had to drop the weights, what I was pleased about though was how much stronger my arms are. I can now do 'fly's' with 7kg in each hand, only a few sessions ago I was doing it with 4kg. I love having strong arms.

I have good news, I gained a distinction in my Open University exam, Sports and Exercise Psychology. My standards are so high that I would have felt like I'd failed without the distinction - the pressure I put myself under! I set myself impossibly high standards, and beat myself up when I don't achieve them.

Friday, 24 June 2011

Oh dear. Finished off the bottle of wine and ate quite a few nuts, this is not a good day! I did a spinning class for the first time yesterday. I enjoyed it but it's hard to judge performance. I wish the bikes had a dial. I tried to push myself and found it hard to cycle up hill at a high setting but I could do it. All of the strength and power my squats have built up was definitely coming into play. The worst part was sitting down, it hurt my bottom!

Have you been watching *Embarrassing Fat Bodies*? Alongside the truly obese there are people who have lost lots of weight through a gastric band or bypass. The difference between them and me is that I've been doing weight bearing exercise which is helping to firm up my skin. I'm now doing arm exercises raising 10kg dumb bells in each arm, and my biceps are now developing, I can actually feel my muscles. My legs are strong too. I do believe it's essential to do weights in addition to dieting. Cardio alone is not enough. I'm never going to get a washboard stomach but I will get as close as I can.

WEEK 92

Monday, 11 July 2011
Weight: 12 stone 5lbs
92lbs total loss, 2lb gain

Yesterday I was training with Emma. Next to us, Pete was training his client - we are the 2 biggest losers at the gym! The guy was amazed at how much weight I had lost and commented that I hadn't lost it from my boobs, Emma told him yes I had and I had had enormous boobs in the past. He also commented on how I was shapely and went in and out, and had a nice bottom. Quite nice to get compliments.

I was so pleased to get on the scales on Friday and I see that I had only put on 1 pound, although I've been eating left overs since our party on Saturday and I could yet gain another pound this week. In addition, we are going to the 2000 Trees Festival and it is always hard to eat healthily when you have to buy food from stalls but I will take nuts and tomatoes and apples so that will be good.

At our party on Saturday people were again amazed at my size. Helen kept on commenting on the lack of fat on my back and some of my male friends were grabbing me around the waist. I didn't pull away!

THE PLATEAU

As we lose weight we need less food to maintain our size, so we need to eat less and exercise more. It can reach a point where it is very hard to do any more. It's easier to lose weight when we are young, rather than to end up struggling in midlife, but as I have shown, it is never too late!

Wednesday, 13 July 2011

Not going great, I have family staying. There is a cupboard full of food left over from our party and it is far too tempting, I've been eating cake, drinking beer and eating pork pie but I have still been going to the gym which is a positive.

Thursday, 14 July 2011

I'm off to another festival later today so went to the gym this morning, I knew I'd have so much to do, including talking with a journalist at 11am. I simply didn't have time for a full hour. So this time I decided to do 2 x 6 minute running sessions, up from 5 minutes, and then do some brisk walking for a further 30 minutes.

WEEK 92

Monday, 18 July 2011
Weight: 12 stone 5lbs
92lbs total loss

Yesterday I went to the gym and again did 2 x 6 minute running sessions and I also walked up hill at 10% incline 5.5kph for 50 minutes. My hamstrings still ache today. I had potato and a Yorkshire pudding with my lunch, followed by cake and wine. I don't think this was the good day I had planned.

Today I will get back on track. For breakfast I had egg and bacon, then a session at the gym with Emma. Today she made me run for 8 minutes, it was hard going but I did it, she wants me to get into running as this is something that I can do from home. After my workout I had a protein shake and at mid day an apple.

I feel quite down at the moment and a lot of this can be attributed to the fact that I am a perfectionist, I beat myself up as I think I could have done so many things better than I have. This covers everything I do from relating to people, to hosting a party or even just writing an article. I've always set myself high standards but it is much worse now and it's really getting in the way. I've no idea why I feel like this.

Wednesday, 20 July 2011

In yesterday's Times newspaper there's an article - 'How to get a bikini body in 2 weeks'. This title might sell papers but how can you possibly make a change in 2 weeks? People want to believe a quick fix will work. It does make me laugh when I read about how it is possible to get Pippa Middleton's bottom in 4 weeks with a few lunges - I do lunges with 7kg in each hand!

Yesterday I had a very busy day with clients but still got to the gym, although today I had a backlog of work. I've been doing a lot of cardio and it has been 18 days since I last did a proper weights session due to knee problems.

Today I felt tired so I skipped the running and instead did more on the cross trainer at level 6. Emma had eaten a big bar of chocolate last night, showing that lots of people slip, that's normal. It's about not falling into the habit of doing it every day and not having lots of different treats and extra helpings.

Emma was telling me that one of her clients can't get over how firm my body is, and she was telling her husband that I'd lost so much weight yet looked nothing like the people on TV who have had a gastric band.

Sunday, 24 July 2011

I'm writing the second edition of *How To Get A Job In A Recession* and writing always makes me want to eat chocolate, how can I break this pattern? I had ham salad for tea, and in the evening ate cheese and crackers, so I'm not too pleased with myself. I also ate rich tea biscuits. I found a bottle of cava in the fridge and drank most of the bottle myself last night, I do love my sparkling wine! I would normally have shared it with Simon but he had been to the pub and had 4 pints, 'you've had enough, this is mine' I told him. This coming week I need to be very focused.

WEEK 97

Monday, 15 August 2011
Weight: 12 stone 11lbs
86lbs total loss, gain!!!

I haven't weighed myself for several weeks, once again I lost my focus. After seeing the gain I'm once again very frustrated with myself but the answer lies within, I know why it has happened: too much of the wrong food and especially too much alcohol. I've just been doing what I want without thinking about the consequences.

WEEK 99

Monday, 29 August 2011
Weight: 13 stone
84lbs total loss, gain

It's my birthday today and we had another party which meant more tempting foods. What a birthday, getting on the scales and finding that once again I'm up to 13 stone. I know a good 2-3lbs of this can be put down to water retention from a lack of food or drink yesterday but it is still so frustrating to be up here again. Not so long ago I was very happy to be back at 12 stone 3. I don't think I will ever get to 11 stone 3. Originally this was my dream target, to be half the woman I was but I now realise that this goal is unrealistic, if I can't maintain 12 stone 3 how can I stay at a stone lighter?

Friday, 2 September 2011

For weeks I've been unfocused. I've eaten good food during the day but in the evenings I've been eating chocolate and drinking wine - often 100g of chocolate and half a bottle of wine in a sitting. Recently I had a family weekend and party and ate bread, cake, trifle and even more wine.

Being strict for 4 days means I have lost 7lbs. I'd planned on a carb meal on Saturday but decided to go for it on Friday, there was half a bottle of wine open in the fridge so I drank that and polished off the rest of the chocolate biscuits. Well they have gone now!

WEEK 101

Monday, 12 September 2011
Weight: 12 stone 5lbs (92lbs total loss)

A good result on the scales, I've lost 9lb in 2 weeks.

'The difference between a successful person and others is not a lack of strength, not a lack of knowledge, but rather in a lack of will.'

Vince Lombardi

A s you have read this you will have seen me repeatedly tell myself that 'This is it, I will lose the rest of my weight to hit my goal'. Time and time again, however, I have instead succumbed to alcohol, chocolate and cheese and biscuits. Many times I told myself that I looked good enough and it was okay to lighten up and have what I wanted but then I put the pounds back on. I then beat myself up, refocused and lost them again. I was trapped in a cycle.

I was losing the same few pounds over and over again. I didn't think I was yo-yo dieting as it was only a few pounds in question, actually 11 pounds as I bounced between 12 stone 03 and 13 stone, but looking back, I now think this has been a wasted year. I feel I let myself down. I'm a perfectionist and I want to do things right.

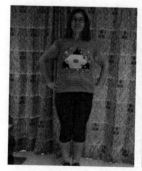
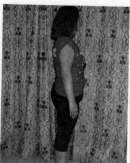
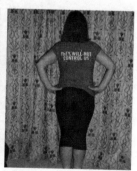

> **You have to want it enough - that's what set me back before.**

As I write this chapter I'm more sanguine, and I think my progress is typical of most people. If I'd gone through and lost all the weight without getting sidetracked you might have felt that my story was an impossible one for you to follow, I've been just as fallible as anyone else but I've still made great progress.

EMMA

That's what I love about you chick, that you pick yourself up and get back on and do it again, and this time we'll lose that last bit of fat and you will be even more awesome than you are now.

Looking back through my diary, I weighed 12 stone 05 on 12 September, 12 stone 09 on Tuesday 27 September, 12 stone 09 on 13th October and hit 13 stone on 22 October. I was writing and then publishing the 2nd edition of *How to Get a Job in a Recession*. Writing a second edition was just as big a task as writing a book from scratch and as with every book there are problems and delays. It took 3 weeks from publishing to getting the book sold on Amazon and the process was very stressful so I returned to my favourite way of dealing with the stress - eating and drinking. I associate writing with eating.

Emma has consistently encouraged me to turn my diary into a book (the one you're reading) but I have kept putting the task off. I wanted to end on a high note, and this high note just hasn't been forthcoming. When *How to Get a Job in a Recession* went on sale, I stopped feeling stressed and I got my focus back. Emma had a plan. I was going to shake up my eating and try a different approach.

WEEK 106

17th October 2011

A new workout today which you can see in the appendix. It was very tough going.

EMMA

Well done today chick for digging in and getting the job done when you felt low! I know I seem harsh sometimes but it's just coz I know what you can do and that you'll feel better once you've done it! X x

The low carb diet was perfect for me when I had a lot of weight to lose, it stopped me being insulin resistant and lead to a great weight loss, but Emma said that I was drawn to alcohol and crackers because my body was craving carbs. My new plan includes regular good carbs with most of my meals. Good carbs include measured quantities of gluten free oats, brown rice or quinoa or sweet potato and banana plus green vegetables. I'm going to start on Sunday.

WEEK 107

Monday, 24 October 2011
Weight: 13 stone
83lbs total loss, gain

Today I made significant changes to my eating and exercise. Things have slipped: I've been eating too much, partly in response to the stress of getting my latest book ready. I've also been unable to exercise properly due to my recurring knee injury.

This new eating plan is a radical departure from my old one. I can eat carbs with almost every meal, I have to weigh all my food very carefully and eat every three hours. The quantities below are based on my current weight and level of exercise and have been carefully worked out by Emma. I've included them so you can get an idea for the quantity of food I can eat and still lost weight. Do remember though that I work out most days, probably burning about 500 calories each time I go to the gym. The amount you would eat may be different.

New Eating Plan

06.30	Before Gym	Triple espresso and large glass of water
07.00-08.00		GYM
09.15	Meal 1	60 grams gluten free oats 100 grams banana 30 grams protein powder
12.15	Meal 2	126 grams (uncooked weight) chicken 30 grams uncooked brown rice 100 grams green beans
15.15	Meal 3	170 grams Salmon fillet (or tuna steak) 210 grams sweet potato (flesh only) 100 grams broccoli
18.15	Meal 4	60 grams gluten free oats 100 grams banana 30 grams protein powder
21.15	Meal 5	3 egg omelette (3 whites, 1 yolk) fried in coconut oil 2 dessert spoons of full fat cottage cheese
22.30	Meal 6	30 grams protein shake OR 10-15 grams walnuts or almonds OR 1 boiled egg and 2 dessert spoons cottage cheese

When Emma told me what to eat I could not see how this would work, there is so much food! I wanted to adapt it and to eat less. Emma told me to trust her, however.

If I understand correctly, my body has not had enough top quality nutrients and so it's been hanging onto fat, so the new eating plan is going to shock my body and after a month or so Emma will reduce the portion sizes.

When I first started on this journey I was eating six meals a day, but I gradually drifted away from this. It's time to return, with a vengeance!

HOW MUCH DOES A PIECE OF CHICKEN WEIGH?

Chicken (and salmon) loses a lot of weight when cooked. For example, cook 540 grams of chicken and once it is cooked in foil it only weighs 420 grams. To begin I weighed out cooked weight but then moved onto basing my figures on food's uncooked weight. Our bodies need 2000 calories a day to run but often the calories we put in ourselves are crap! If I think about the total number of calories I've consumed on top of 'good calories' - a couple of slices of toast, cheese and biscuits, ice cream, half a bottle of wine – then I see that I've been consuming far more calories than the 2,000 I should have.

Saturday, 29 October 2011

I've started my new diet and I feel ill – could this partly be down to caffeine withdrawal? I was drinking quite a lot of coffee throughout the day but now I've cut down to just a couple of cups in the morning. I had to skip the gym for a couple of days due to illness but I'm now feeling so full of energy, Emma says it's the carb boost!

My gym week now includes two days of weights with Emma in addition to 4 cardio sessions which I do on my own.

WE CAN FIND TIME TO EXERCISE

It's too easy to convince ourselves that we don't have time for the gym, but if something is important we can always make the time. When I go to the gym at 6.30am it's full of people who prioritise and work out before work. Working for myself allows me to to put gym visits in my diary and fit my work around these.

WEEK 108

Monday, 31 October 2011
Weight: 12 stone 7lbs
90lbs total loss

One week on and I've lost 7lbs, I truly am amazed. Simon can't believe how much I'm eating but it is all high quality food, not one ounce of rubbish. I'm now totally committed to following this plan for a total of 8 weeks.

I think I've got my weight loss mojo back and I am so focused. I'm imagining the feeling of being able to tell people that I've lost over 145lbs (10 stone 7 pounds). In the long term I'm still going to strive to be half the woman I was as my stretch goal.

I took a dress back to a store. When I told the sales assistant that it made me look pregnant she said, 'you don't want that, you are so skinny!' I still don't think they are describing me when I hear comments like this.

**ALL THESE YEARS OF BEING UNHAPPY AND
EMBARRASSED, NOW I LOVE LIFE**

I thought I would die fat - through my 30s and 40s I've been fat. I pretended I didn't mind, all the while looking for the quick fix. So many times I would start a diet and then give up, many times because I didn't see a drop on the scales. I could get down thinking of how I missed out during the best years of my life, but now I look to the future, no longer apologising for my size. I want to get out there and I am proud of who I am. I've now found the inner confident self that has been hiding from me for so long.

Wednesday, 2 November 2011

I've got so much energy! Emma told me I would and I didn't believe her. I'm exercising every day. I do weights twice a week and I spend the rest of the week mainly going to the gym to do cardio and if I don't make it to the gym then I go for a brisk walk.

My new eating plan allows me to eat a 'cheat' meal once a week. This means that I eat my food as normal but can add in something extra. We were out for a meeting with Skeptics in the Pub and were all having a Thai buffet. I didn't realise that the buffet food brought out was just the starter, and I ate more than I would have if I'd known we were also getting a main meal each. But I enjoyed every mouthful and I also kept away from the alcohol. I'm wondering if I should abstain from alcohol, I feel so much better each morning waking up without having drank the night before. Plus, alcohol is not part of this plan.

I had eaten so much I didn't want to eat my eggs or nuts when I got home. Checking with Emma, I should have eaten these meals even if I wasn't hungry. It was the first time I've made this mistake so I've learned for the future.

> **EATING CLEAN**
>
> A real benefit of eating clean is that I don't want alcohol. I feel so good inside that I don't want to do anything that will upset my inner balance.

Sunday, 6 November 2011

I was at a conference this weekend and I planned in advance for this. I could have decided to go off plan, but my commitment to my goal was more important than appearing odd! This time I took my own food with me, I packed up a cool box with all the food I needed. I don't mind eating my meals cold.

On Saturday I ate my oats mix when I arrived, had my chicken meal for my lunch with the other delegates, went to my room and ate my salmon meal in the afternoon tea break, ate oats before dinner and then had the conference dinner - steak, green beans and fruit salad as my 'cheat meal'. On Sunday I had oats in my room, had my chicken meal for lunch with the other delegates and ate my salmon meal at the end of the conference.

I was very pleased to have kept my focus, if I'd decided that I'd go off plan it might have been harder to get back on track. I'm only 2 weeks into this plan and we go on holiday in 6 weeks, so that's my deadline.

WEEK 109

Monday, 7 November 2011
Weight: 12 stone 5 lbs
92lb total loss

A 2 pound loss - result!

I've had a lot of problems with my knee and this has stopped me doing the sorts of exercises that use up fat and helps tone up my bottom and legs. I'm now wearing a knee support and since 19 October I'm once again doing the type of exercises I like.

My new programme involves squats holding a weight. I started with 10kg and today I moved up to 14kg. I'm also doing chest fly's with 7kg and 'Russian twists' with a medicine ball, moving up from 6kg to 7kg. I then do walking lunges and have moved up from doing this with 6kg to doing this with 8kg. I get a short break and move onto push presses holding a weight, starting with 6kg and moving up to 9 kg. (I bend with the weight at bust level then as I come up I lift the weight above my head, I do this 25 times in each set). I then do chest press laying on a Swiss Ball with 9kg in each hand, and then a couple of exercises using machines - the seated row and quad extensions. These second ones are so tough but I've moved up from doing 20 at 20kg to doing 20 at 35kg. A Fitness Instructor would be able to show you how to do these and the other exercises I do.

ZONE OUT

Some exercises are tough. It is easy to tell our selves that we can't do something. What helps is to find a 'happy place' inside so you don't focus on the pain and just keep going.

Tuesday, 8 November 2011

Family from overseas came to visit today. I wondered what I should give them to eat so that we could all eat together, I decided on roast chicken and green beans. They had baked potatoes, I had cold brown rice. They hadn't seen me for ages and couldn't believe my weight loss - but it's true, I have done it.

Friday, 11 November 2011

Yesterday I went to London, I was guest speaker at the Career Writers Association meeting. I took my own food with me and ate oats on the train and ate my chicken meal on the tube. The meeting ran longer than I expected as they asked so many questions. I went to see a client, then ate my salmon meal on the return train journey. I'd bought some plastic food containers that were all the same size which meant as I finished a meal I could stack them up for the journey home.

I'm so happy I can't stop smiling! My mood is stable and this change of diet is just what I needed. I now wish I'd made the change this time last year, but maybe it was important for me to go through a time of struggle so that I would be ready to return with such a thirst for success!

WEEK 110

Tuesday, 15 November 2011
Weight: 12 stone 03
94lb total loss

We have the cover photo shoot (for this book) on Friday and Emma wants me looking as good as possible. She adapted my diet and for Thursday - Sunday I was on half carbs, everything else stayed the same but I only ate half the usual amount of oats, rice and sweet potato. It has been tough, I've got used to a higher quantity of food.

I got on the scales today and I've lost another two pounds. In 3 weeks I've lost 11 pounds and I'm pleased, if I can lose a pound a week from now on then that would be perfect. I feel different this time, this time I think the weight loss will be sustainable and I think I have finally broken free from the trappings of my yo-yo approach.

Spent time doing more cardio at the gym, had one client session and then spent the rest of the day working on this book. I do put extra pressure on myself. I want to get this book complete and in the shops as soon as possible. This evening we booked a table at the Jamaican night at Storyteller, a Cheltenham restaurant. The first item on the menu was a Pina Colada, followed by Jerk chicken with hot sauce and pineapple salsa, then Red Stripe beer followed by Goat curry with rice and beans, oven proof rum and ginger beer, then sweet potato and coconut tart with ice cream and finally rum and carrot juice. I'd committed to giving up alcohol till our holiday so decided that Simon would drink all the alcohol, he didn't complain and I just sniffed the alcohol, not quite as good but thankfully I stayed firm!

WEEK 111

Friday, 18 November 2011

Today was the photo shoot and Emma and I had a brilliant time. I worked out with Emma at the gym on Wednesday and spent the majority of the day writing this book. Yesterday and this morning has been a little different, Emma ordered me NOT to exercise and to rest, to leave all thoughts of work to one side. This has been so hard and, strangely, it has made me tired. Yesterday I went and bought some new bras and again spoke to the sales assistant about how different I feel having lost the weight and about how much I like the new me. Today I weigh 12 stone and 2 pounds which is brilliant, especially considering that I haven't exercised for 2 days. With 4 weeks till our holiday I'll easily crack the 12 stone barrier before we go away.

We parked close to the studio and I got a little confused over the parking ticket, a young man ran after me as I'd forgotten to collect it. He handed it over and said 'you are one hot lady, want a date?' I think he was about 25, I told him I was married, it was flattering to be asked. It really was, I'm not used to being chatted up, I honestly can't remember the last time, it was so long ago. I was looking good and very excited after the photos. I think I radiated happiness and confidence, Simon had better watch out!

WEEK 112

Monday, 21 November 2011
Weight: 12 stone 01
96lb total loss

12 stone 1, tantalisingly close to breaking through the 12 stone barrier. Another good session with Emma at the gym, and a very focused work day as well.

Wednesday, 23 November 2011

Gosh sometimes it is tough to do that bit more. Today when I had to increase my reps from 25 to thirty, I said ' hurty, thirty'. But you have to push yourself, you can't think what you did last time is enough because that's one sure way to plateau.

I continue to drink lots of water. Drinking a litre for every 50 pounds of body weight means that at 12 stone I need to drink over 3 litres (over 5 pints) every day and this is in addition to the water I drink at the gym.

Newspapers are full of stories of people who lost weight through gastric bands and gastric bypasses. There are hardly any stories about people who do it naturally like me. I think it's because it takes much longer, but the benefits are that we don't then have excess skin which needs to be removed. Recently I read about a lady who paid £5,000 to have a gastric band fitted but then she was left with excess skin. To remove this cost her £14,000 for a body lift and she spent a further £16,000 on arm, breast and thigh lifts. That's £35,000 pounds! I could have personal training sessions, twice a week for 10 years for that price and I'd be naturally toned.

Friday, 25 November 2011

I've stayed focused with both my food and exercise. As I read through this chapter I'm feeling great about how I continue to push myself further at the gym. Chest flys, where you open arms wide and bring the weights into the chest, have increased from 7kg to 10 kg; I'm doing Russian twists with 10kg, I started with 6kg, I do walking lunges with 12kg and had started with 6kg and the quad extensions have gone up from 20kg to 40kg.

Saturday, 26 November 2011

Recently I've bought quite a lot of clothes. As I dropped down the sizes I looked to buy cheap clothes. When I was very fat I had to buy expensive clothes, the cheap larger sizes were in polyester, I wanted flattering well cut clothes so I bought clothes from an expensive Italian mail order company. Now I can buy low cost chain store clothes, but I've also treated myself to 3 beautiful dresses - a flapper beaded dress from Jigsaw, a bodycon dress from Reiss and today a full length white fitted beaded dress. This is absolutely beautiful and I plan to wear it on New Years Eve. It's a good fit and will still look good if I lose a further 7 pounds, but I don't want to gain any weight! I chatted with Simon and said this is my incentive to stay at this weight.

WEEK 113

Monday, 28 November 2011
Weight: 12 stone 00
97lb total loss

I've lost 2 pounds a week for the last 3 weeks and was really hoping to get the same today. Just a pound though. It doesn't sound much, but it still makes a difference.

I have worked so hard at eating correctly and I've been cramming exercise into every spare moment of this past week. It's been tough and I've done more than usual but every now and again it is great to really push forward. I'm so pleased with my new eating programme, I love the return to regular eating and it is making me feel great. Before today's strength session, Emma checked my measurements. It's been ages since we have done this. There really wasn't any point when the scales were fluctuating. I was looking forward to seeing what the final measurements for the book would be. Although I'm only one pound lighter than the last time we measured on 20th June, over the past 5 months I've continued to exercise. The chart below shows my measurements at my fattest, when I started 2 years, ago, for June and finally, for today.

	At my fattest	09/10/09	20/6/11	28/11/11
Bust	156	136.5	100	100
Biceps, right	47.5	36	25.6	25
Waist	154	133	93	92.5
Hips	155	138.5	104	102
Thigh- right	80	67	53	52.5
Thigh- left	76.5	71.5	58	57
Calves - right	50.5	47.5	39	39
Calves - left	52		40	39

You can see below the overall drop in cms from my fattest.

Bust	From 156cm to 100. A loss of 56cm
Biceps, right	From 47.5cm to 24.5. A loss of 23 cm
Waist	From 154cm to 92.5cm. A loss of 61.5cm
Hips	From 155cm to 102cm. A loss of 53cm
Thigh, right	From 80cm to 52.5cm. A loss of 27.5cm
Thigh, left	From 76.5cm to 57cm. A loss of 18.5cm
Calf, right	From 50.5cm to 39cm. A loss of 11.5 cm
Calf, left	From 52cm to 39cm. A loss of 13cm

We followed this with a new exercise programme, I'd stayed on my last one longer than normal. Once again, time to shake my body up. As always, it was hard going as my body got used to doing new things.

Tuesday, 29th November 2011

The season is changing; it's turning to winter and it was cold and dark when I was getting up this morning, but I did it, had my coffee and then got to the gym before 7. I spent 10 minutes on the cross trainer, 10 minutes on the bike and then walked up hill at an 8% incline for 40 minutes. I like my return to uphill walking, it is very satisfying and I also find that I can think while doing it. When I'm lifting weights I have to concentrate.

Sunday, 4th December 2011

I have been really focused this week and I made sure that I went to the gym every day.

I also found the time for a couple of 20 minute walks each day. Actually, I went running each day, and I really am running now, not just jogging. I don't plan to run for long distances but it feels great to be able to run for 10 minutes and then do a brisk walk back. I've had a great week and can't wait to get on the scales tomorrow to do my final weigh in for this book.

I've now completed 6 weeks of this eating plan and drank no alcohol for 6 weeks. I haven't missed it at all and I have lots of energy thanks to a great diet and decent sleep. This week I've really pushed my exercise regime: I worked out with weights on Monday and Wednesday, followed by 20 minutes spent walking on an 8% incline. The other days at the gym I have walked for 60 minutes on an incline, progressing to an incline of 10% today - an hour of walking at 10%! - but hey, I can do it, so ever onwards.

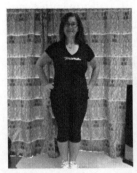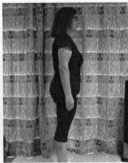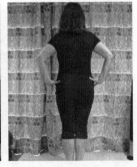

Waking up this morning I smile. Twenty four brand new hours are before me. I vow to life fully in each moment and look at all beings with eyes of compassion.

- Thich Nhat Hanh

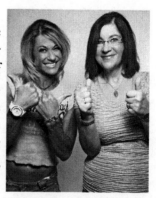

Today is 5th December, this is the last diary entry I can write in order to still meet the publication date of this book. I've kept my focus and for 6 weeks I've been carefully eating everything Emma has told me to. When she first started me on carbs and 2000 calories a day I could not believe that it would make such a difference, but it has.

In 6 weeks I've lost just over a stone. Staying focused leads to brilliant rewards and I've crashed through the 12 stone barrier - 11 stone 12.

This is not just a story of losing weight, but of gaining fitness and regaining confidence - I truely am a new woman, both inside and out.

It's the change inside which is the most amazing change. I am now so confident, so happy and I can't stop smiling. I know that this time my weight loss is sustainable. I now love who I am, love what I can do, and know this change will last forever. My clients have always said I'm amazing, yes, I am!

This is not the end, I will continue to maintain my new state of health and fitness. I've already set myself some new goals including to do the 3 peaks challenge and perhaps Mount Kilimanjaro?

To keep up to date you can read my blog or Like my Facebook page.

If this book has inspired you to make a change to your health, do make your commitment known on Facebook, I'd love to see you make progress too!

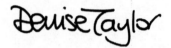

www.fat2fantastic.com

http://www.facebook.com/Fat2Fantastic

www.twitter.com/fat2fantastic

My diary helped keep me focused and motivated and I sincerely hope it will inspire you.

It's not about being skinny, but developing a healthy relationship with food, eating good food, exercising more and believing that you can make a change.

You are so much more than what you read on the scales. You are a wonderful human being no matter what size you are. Loving who we are is a great first step to treating ourselves well.

I am developing materials to enable people just like you to start on your own journey from FAT to fantastic and to be by your side as you have setbacks. Signing up via the **FAT2fantastic.com** website will ensure you are kept informed and receive helpful hints and tips.

Sign up at _www.fat2fantastic.com_

I've already got some tip sheets ready to send on covering both food and exercise and more will be on its way to you over the coming weeks.

You can also join me on Facebook /Fat2Fantastic and post comments and ask questions. Here I'll post short links to interesting articles and short updates.

You can also read my blog, I'll be writing each week as I continue to maintain my loss and work on my next health goals.

START TODAY

Starting today you can choose to move more. It doesn't have to be the gym, just go for a walk, and with a pedometer you can log your progress and move that bit more week on week. Later you may decide to go to a gym, but you could also join a walking group, a dance class or go swimming. It's more important to choose something that you will enjoy.

A personal trainer may be beyond your budget, but perhaps you have a friend who can motivate you to do that bit more. Yes, I worked out with Emma, but it was me who lifted the weight and got me to the gym, week after week.

Log your food, and be truthful. I've shared the huge amount of food I ate before I started my journey, and seeing it written down helped me decide to make a change.

BE IN IT FOR THE LONG TERM

It's taken me years but I got there, one day at a time. Each day I ate well and moved more was helping me move towards my long term goal. As you have read I've had many setbacks but eventually reached my goal and I'm sure you will too.

Wishing you all the very best

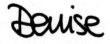

ACKNOWLEDGEMENTS

I would never have started this weight loss diary without the encouragement of Ben Carpenter. It was his knowledge and support that got me focused, he planted the notion that this time I could succeed, which grew into this success story.

Emma continued to support me as I adhered to my food and exercise plan. She's moved from being my personal trainer to a close friend. She knows me oh so well. You can't lie to a PT.

Simon - I love you more now than ever. I don't know how you have put up with me over the years. You've supported me through the low periods, and the mood swings. You've gone along with my eating plan and eating more veggies than you ever thought possible. Yes, you now eat sprouts because I wanted you healthy too.

My friends and colleagues who continued to praise me for my achievements, Facebook has been brilliant in allowing friends all round the world to tell me how great I look and provide the reinforcement that makes me want to continue. I'd particularly like to acknowledge my family - Valerie, Julie and John, Natalie, Jim and Mary, Nick and Natalie, Sarah and Dan for telling me I look amazing and making sure I wasn't tempted by offering me the wrong foods.

I've had brilliant feedback from the trainers at my gym, and complimentary comments from so many other gym members but I can't remember your names, sorry.

Clients, colleagues, neighbours - you know who you are, and I loved the way each time you saw me you told me how well I was doing.

As I wrote the book I used 5 critical readers who have helped to make this an even better book. Thanks to Clare Coyle, Helen Willoughby, Kathryn Pepper, Lucy Herrett and Lisa Ledster. I appreciated each and every piece of feedback you provided. Lucy, I can still hear in my head - but how did it make you feel?

Finally, thanks to Drew Cameron, my editor for ensuring this reads well, Paul Ennis for proof reading and Tudor Maier, for the fantastic layout and cover.

The photo shoot took place at Revolve Studio, Cheltenham. Hair by Holly Palmer, Makeup by Josie Evans, Photos by Ben Durbridge and Dean Dode, photo finishing by Simon Spencer. Thanks to you all.

KEY PRINCIPLES OF THE PALEO DIET

This is the way I ate for the first 9 months and then gradually lightened up, and the weight loss stalled! It is based around eating unprocessed food.

- **Eating clean:** This means avoiding all food that can put stress on the body - alcohol, sugar, coffee, tea, fizzy drinks, chemical additives like aspartame and food colouring, and also dairy, wheat and gluten.

- **Water:** Drink 1 litre of water for every 50lb of body weight. This helps to rid our body of toxins.

- **Drink green tea, and tulsi tea:** These are low or free of caffeine. Green tea can boost our metabolism.

- **Eat protein with every meal:** It stabilises blood sugar, prevents hunger and fuels our muscles.

- **Eat real food:** Not processed, not diet foods. If the packaging contains ingredients we haven't heard of, avoid them.

- **Eat enough food:** If we go on a low calorie diet we may lose weight quickly but this is not necessarily fat and could well be muscle.

- **Don't count calories:** All calories are not the same. You could eat a handful of nuts or a chocolate bar. One has vitamins, minerals and good fats. The other contains few nutrients.

- **Eat 6 or 7 meals a day** - I was told that the quantities were not important but always to sit down to eat. Also to eat 6 or 7 times a day and never go for more than 3 hours before eating again.

It's not focused on a vegetarian diet, but can probably be adapted. All food to be cooked conventionally, not microwaved. Our body needs to be fuelled, we then get a sustained release of energy throughout the day and don't get the late afternoon energy drop. It's not 7 large meals but our food divided into smaller meals.

- **Meat**: Beef, Chicken, Turkey, Lamb, Wild Game, Pork (if free range).

- **Fish**: Salmon, Tuna, Sardines.

- **Fruit** : Berries, Apples, Pears. Other fruit is higher in fructose which can raise blood sugar.

- **Vegetables:** Artichoke, Asparagus, Avocado, Broccoli, Brussel sprouts, Cabbage (green and red), Carrots, Cauliflower, Celery, Chicory, Chinese cabbage, Chives, Courgettes, Cucumber, Endive, Fennel, Garlic, Green beans, Kale, Kohlrabi, Lettuce (avoid iceberg), Mushrooms, Mustard & Cress, Onions, Parsley, Peppers (all kinds), Plantain, Radish, Seaweed, Spinach, Swiss chard, Tomatoes, Turnips, Watercress.

- **Nuts:** Almonds, Walnuts, Pecans - not roasted.

- **Seeds:** Pumpkins, Sunflower.

- **Eggs:** Free Range.

- **Herbs and Spices:** Cinnamon is excellent as it increased the production of insulin and thus helps us to lose fat.

- **Healthy Fats:** Olive or walnut oil for salad dressings and to cook with Coconut oil or Palm oil.

- **Sugar:** Sugar (including artificial sweeteners and honey) triggers the reward centre in our brain and makes us want more sweet things. It really can interfere with our will power.

- **Dairy:** Milk, cheese, yoghurt, ice-cream. **Low fat milk** raises blood sugar levels. The pasteurisation treatment kills the enzymes we need to digest milk.

- **Processed foods, including diet foods:** Cereal, bread, cake, biscuits, pastries, anything with a list of ingredients we don't understand or can't pronounce.

- **Grains:** Wheat, Oats, Barley.

- Potatoes, Parsnip, Pumpkin, Corn.

- **Legumes:** Peanuts.

- **Fizzy diet drinks:** Carbonation introduces carbon dioxide into our body and diet drinks swaps sugar for artificial sweeteners and leads to cravings for carbs.

- **Caffeine:** This puts stress on our body and should be avoided or kept to just 1 cup a day before going to the gym. It leads to over excitement, and a need for sugary foods.

- **Alcohol:** This is a toxin and puts a strain on our liver, kidneys and other vital organs. It triggers insulin secretion and increases body fat storage. It contains empty calories, no nutritional benefits and draws water out of our cells.

- Dried fruit.

- Canned food except tinned tomatoes.

- Hydrogenated margarine and Processed oils.

DAY	Breakfast with fish oil	Mid morning	Lunch	Mid afternoon	Dinner	Mid evening	EXERCISE
MON	½ juiced cucumber; Cooked tomatoes & smoked mackerel	Protein shake	Smoked mackerel and huge plate of salad	25g almonds	Sea bass and broccoli	Protein shake Frozen blueberries	Strength training with Emma
TUES	½ juiced cucumber; Fried egg, bacon and 100g mushrooms	Protein shake, ½ slice ham, 5 cherry tomatoes	Turkey and huge plate of salad	25g almonds juiced cucumber	Plaice, very large piece and broccoli	Slice of turkey and tomatoes; portion of strawberries	1 hour cardio
WED	½ juiced cucumber; Fried egg, 2 slices bacon, 1/2 tin of tomatoes	Protein shake	2 x chicken thighs and large plate of salad	Slice of turkey and tomatoes	Roast chicken and roasted vegetables, cooked in coconut oil	Portion of nuts Protein shake Frozen blueberries	Strength training with Emma
THURS	½ juiced cucumber; Scrambled eggs and mushrooms	25g almonds	Roll mop herring with a large plate of salad	Apple Slice of turkey and tomatoes	Pheasant casserole, extra green beans Portion of nuts	Beef casserole; portion of strawberries	Walk to shop, carried 13lb of shopping on return journey
FRI	½ juiced cucumber; Smoked mackerel	Protein shake	Huge plate of salad with ham and small amount of feta cheese	2 slices of turkey	Salmon and green beans 2 squares divine chocolate	Carrot batons and houmous; frozen blueberries	1 hour cardio
SAT	½ juiced cucumber; Scrambled eggs and bacon	Protein shake	Steak and huge plate of salad	25g almonds	Beef casserole and cabbage	3 slices of turkey; apple; protein shake	Strength training at the gym
SUN	½ juiced cucumber; 2 fried eggs, 2 slices bacon and 1/2 tin of tomatoes	25g almonds	Beef casserole and cabbage	Carrot batons and houmous	Ribs of beef, sprouts, carrots, roast potatoes, large glass of wine and slice of cheesecake	Carrot batons and houmous	Walk up Bredon Hill

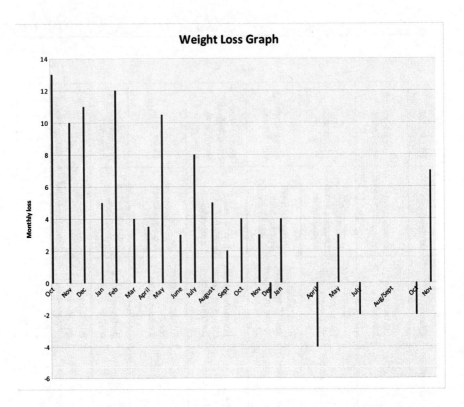

We are lead to believe we will have a regular weight loss, but as you can see above there were drops in monthly weight loss even in the earlier months

Oct 0	13	Aug 10	5
Nov 09	10	Sept 10	2
Dec 09	11	Oct 10	4
Jan 10	5	Nov 10	3
Feb 10	12	Dec 101	-1
Mar 10	4	Jan 11	4
April 10	3.5	April 11	-4
May 10	10.5	May 11	3
June 10	3	July 11	-2
July 10	8		

SAMPLE STRENGTH TRAINING PROGRAMME
BEGINNERS

A1 – step ups from mid shin

12 October (with Ben)	15	15		
13 October	18	19		
15 October (with Ben)	20	20	20	
17 October Higher step	20	20	20	
20 October Higher step	20	20	20	
22 October (with Ben) +3kg	15	15	15	15

A2 – dumb bell row

12 October (with Ben) 8kg	12	15		
13 October	18	19		
15 October (with Ben)	8kg 20	9kg 15	9kg 15	
17 October	20	20	20	
20 October	18	18	18	
22 October (with Ben) 10kg	12	12	12	12

A2 – dumb bell row

12 October (with Ben) 7kg	10	10	12	
13 October	16	15		
15 October (with Ben)	13	13	13	
17 October	16	16	16	
20 October	18	18	18	
22 October (with Ben) 8kg	12	12	12	12

A1 – step ups from mid shin

12 October (with Ben)	7.2	7.2		
13 October	7.2	7.2	7.2	
15 October (with Ben)	7.4	7.4	7.4	
17 October	7.6	7.6	7.4	
20 October	7.8	7.8	7.8	
22 October (with Ben)	8.0	8.0	8.0	8.0

A2 – dumb bell row

12 October (with Ben) 20kg	12	12		
13 October	18	19		
15 October (with Ben) 25kg	15	12	12	
17 October	16	14	14	
20 October	18	20	18	
22 October (with Ben) 30kg	12	12	12	12

A2 – dumb bell row

12 October (with Ben)	12	12		
13 October	14	14		
15 October (with Ben)	20	20	20	
17 October	22	22	22	
20 October	22	22	22	
22 October (with Ben)	26	26	30	26

SAMPLE STRENGTH TRAINING PROGRAMME
ADVANCED

Warm up - Cross trainer 10 minutes, level 4, 130 RPM

		17 Oct	19 Oct	24 Oct	26 Oct	31 Oct	2 Nov	4 Nov	7 Nov
A1	GOBLET SQUAT	10kg 25 x 3	12kg 25 x 3	12kg 30 x 3	12kg 20 x 3	12kg 25 x 3	12kg 25 x 3	14kg 25 x 3	16kg 25 x 3
A2	CHEST FLYS	7kg 20 x 3	7kg 20 x 3	7kg 20 x 3	7kg 20 x 3	7kg 20 x 3	7kg 20 x 3	7kg 20 x 3	8kg 20 x 3
A3	RUSSIAN TWIST	6kg 40 x 3	6kg 40 x 3	7kg 40 x 3	7kg 40 x 3	7kg 40 x 3	7kg 40 x 3	7kg 40 x 3	8kg 40 x 3
A4	WALKING LUNGES	6kg 24 x 3	7kg 24 x 3	8kg 24 x 3	8kg 24 x 3	8kg 24 x 3	8kg 24 x 3	9kg 12 x 3	9kg 12 x 3
B1	PUSH PRESS	9kg 20 x 3	9kg 25 x 3	9kg 25 x 3	9kg 25 x 3	9kg 25 x 3	9kg 25 x 3	9kg 20 x 3	10kg 25 x 3
B2	CHEST PRESS	8kg 20 x 3	8kg 20 x 3	8kg 20 x 3	8kg 20 x 3	9kg 20 x 3	9kg 20 x 3	9kg 20 x 3	10kg 20 x 3
B3	SEATED ROW	25kg 15 x 3	25kg 20 x 3	25kg 20 x 3	25kg 20 x 3	25kg 20 x 3	25kg 20 x 3	25kg 20 x 3	30kg 15,15,20
B4	QUAD EXTENTION	20kg 20 x 3	20kg 20 x 3	20kg 20 x 3	20kg 20 x 3	20kg 20 x 3	20kg 20 x 3	25 kg 20 x 3	30kg 20 x 3

FURTHER INFORMATION

Follow Denise as she continues through maintenance by reading her blog at *www.FAT2fantastic.com* and *facebook.com/Fat2Fantastic*

FREE STUFF

Access free materials such as food diary templates and downloadable shopping guides through signing up at the website.

MEDIA

Denise is very happy to discuss her story and provide motivational support to your readers. Contact the office on 01684 772888 or 07931 303367.

ADDITIONAL SERVICES

Do you want to go from FAT to Fantastic? A group programme is under development, sign up on the website to be kept informed.

Would you like a personal consultation with Emma? You can email her at *emmabrace669@yahoo.co.uk* or call her on 07710 755596

www.fat2fantastic.com
www.facebook.com/Fat2Fantastic
twitter.com/fat2fantastic

How to Get a Job in a Recession 2012: A Comprehensive Guide to Job Hunting in the 21st Century, Complete with Masses of Free Downloadable Bonuses

Denise Taylor

It's a competitive jobs market and coming second will not get you the job. This revised and updated 2nd edition of How to Get a Job in a Recession provides practical advice with masses of free bonuses in an easy to follow, straightforward guide.

It's like a one-to-one job search coaching session providing expert advice and a structured plan.

This book will be relevant for you whether you are at the start of your career or a job changer who needs both a reminder of the basics and an introduction to the most effective ways to find a job. HINT: it's not sat at your computer all day, nor is it concentrating on jobs you see advertised, that's what everyone else is doing. You will learn how to research and contact companies direct, making effective use of the people you know.

Section 3 guides you through how to find things out with chapters on Networking, Fact-finding interviews and Research for job search.

Section 5: Active Job Search has chapters on the direct approach, targeting the hidden job market, Being found, beyond LinkedIn and radical approaches for you to pick and chose the ones which may work for you.

Too many people fail to get the job they want. They put too much energy into traditional ways of applying for a job. In this dramatically revised 2nd edition you will get a systematic practical guide through all aspects of job search. Learn:

- Why you have to be clear on what you want to do, and how to create a message.

- The importance of research and why you need to go far beyond a review of the company website.
- How to effectively target an application through a customised CV and cover letter.
- Why you must be on LinkedIn and how to use it as part of your job search campaign.
- Why you have to be found and how to do this.
- How to prepare for a Skype interview.
- How to stay motivated.

... And MUCH MORE

Alongside the 23 chapters of practical advice you also get access to:

- Orientation welcome video.
- 20+ forms to download for your own personal use in managing your job hunt.
- 3 audio interviews on Thinking yourself to success, Body language, Using career assessments.
- Mock interview brief to use in your interview practice.
- Easy access to all the web links referred to in the book.

Don't waste another day - get focused on a targeted job search now!

Visit *www.howtogetajobinarecession.com* for more information

Lightning Source UK Ltd.
Milton Keynes UK
UKOW05f2205140414

229984UK00022B/1180/P